The Hopelessly Human Nurse

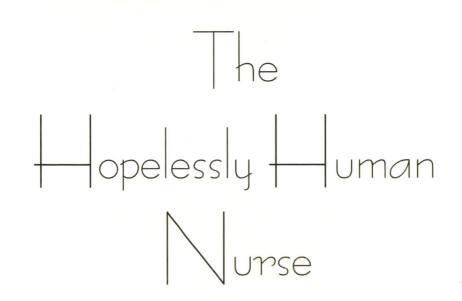

The Hopelessly Human Nurse

a marriage of the
art & science within

Linda Bridge and Kathy Knowles

Published by
Hopelessly Human Productions Inc.
Box 1092, Lethbridge, Alberta, Canada T1J 4A2

Illustrated by Rosalie Wilson, Lethbridge, AB.
Edited by Yvonne Jeffery, Calgary, AB.
Book cover based on the original design by Adair Advertising.
Printed in Canada by The Warwick Printing Co. Ltd., Lethbridge, AB.

Library and Archives Canada Cataloguing in Publication Data:

Bridge, Linda, 1958-

The hopelessly human nurse: a marriage of the art and science within

Linda Bridge & Kathy Knowles

Includes bibliographical references.

ISBN 0-9736040-1-8

1. Nursing.   2. Nursing-Anecdotes.   I. Knowles, Kathy, 1959-   II. Title.

RT82.B746 2006   610.73   C2006-905288-3

This book is intended to serve as a catalyst for positive change. It is not intended to be, and should not be relied upon, as a substitute for competent individual medical, psychiatric, psychological or psycho-therapeutic advice, or other professional counselling. Neither the authors nor the publisher by this book are, or purport to be, engaged in rendering medical, psychiatric, psychological, psycho-therapeutic advice, or are engaged in professional counselling of any nature or kind whatsoever.

The authors and publisher disclaim all responsibility for any claim, loss, damages, or liability, personal or otherwise, howsoever caused or arising, and whether arising or caused directly or indirectly, alleged to have occurred as a result of the use and application of any of the contents of this book.

To the man who said,

"You must each be a lamp unto yourselves."

Siddhartha Gautama

I feel very strongly these days that we are failing to develop the social and humanistic side of nursing — the spirit of nursing as we used to call it — and all that goes to the balancing of the scientific and technical aspects ... I am distressed to realize that we are doing less in this field today than we did a few years ago and there seems to be very little interest in it ... It is a part of the sickness of our civilization that we have over stressed the scientific and technical side and have neglected the other aspects of our work and education.

Isabel M. Stewart (1878 – 1963)
Canadian-born, U. S. nursing scholar and leader

We must learn to live together as brothers or we will perish together as fools. Martin Luther King Jr.

Universe, grant me the courage to accept that I can change, and to embark upon the journey, and the wisdom to understand that my new reflection will change others.

Kathy Knowles

Contents

F. I. P.

Foreword, Introduction and Preface

A wedding is needed with white dresses and dancing and cake. A wedding is necessary with passion and patience and boundaries. A marriage is required with friendship and courage and mistakes. A union is essential with forgiveness and flowers and feelings. A nuptial is desired with intimacy and intuition and analysis. A wedding is needed with fears and assertions and respect.

Nurses have the ability to effectively shift the health care system to a healthier state. No other group in society carries this positive influential power.

I haven't spoken with anyone during this past year of travel who did not know a nurse, either intimately, through a family or friend connection, or via professional exposure. 'Everyone Knows a Nurse' has become a new mantra.

People speak of their innate trust in nurses and the value that they place on our input. There is high regard for our knowledge, caring and respect for human life. Caring for others in their most vulnerable moments makes nurses valuable role models and mentors for our communities and our world.

The respect for my power as a nurse grows deeper daily. What I am reflecting to others affects the world greatly

— more than I ever imagined.

I did not always project my best self — and will display this shortcoming again in the future. I am human — hopelessly human. It is because I am hopelessly human that I know the key that will help unlock the health of the world. The key is me.

I am a valuable human being — a human being of great wealth and merit. Caring for myself with the utmost respect and love, through my thoughts, words and actions, reflects to others. As I value myself as a uniquely special woman and live true to my beliefs, this truth and happiness is mirrored to those around me.

Learning to be my own best friend marries my art and science within. This authenticity allows me to be healthier and happier.

It is a journey of trial and error and new choices — life's lessons viewed from a different angle.

Moving forward with the melding of art and science will lead to an acceptance of self and therefore the world. This shift will tilt the direction of health care allowing it to heal from the inside out. My belief in the ability of nurses to change the system is what propels me to share my thoughts. This is the way. Let the courtship begin.

A wedding is needed and I look forward to the dance.

K. K.

So, a wedding is needed. I wonder what my parents will think of this union — the marriage of my art and science within?

On my fortieth birthday my parents came for a visit, and they arrived with a very large present. Our family did not usually give large presents, so I was intrigued.

They were both grinning from ear to ear with a private joke.

"What's going on?" I asked.

Dad started, "Well, this is your wedding present."

"My what?"

Mom interjected. "Everyone else was given china for their weddings, so we wanted to do the same for you."

"Does this mean you've given up on me? What happens if I get married later?"

Not missing a beat, my mom responded, "Well you'll still need silverware."

This talk of wedding presents has me wondering how I am going to explore and expose my art and science sides, so I can proceed toward marrying the two parts of 'me.'

My assumption was that this had already taken place, and that the two were blissfully coexisting within me. I now realize they had been neither truly married nor blissful.

An awareness of my thoughts and feelings, faults and all, is needed to fully wed my science and art together. Building my self respect allows me to artfully practice the science of nursing.

Touching on my own humanness has been full of falling down, falling off, and climbing back up adventures.

I will no longer sit in a boat simply skimming across the surface of life. I need to dive in and submerse myself in the depths below, to feel the air burning in my lungs. Experiencing the cold, the warmth, the hidden caves and beautiful colors is what I want.

Inconsistent use of my art caused me to focus on my science side. I had not dug deep enough into the what and the why of certain feelings and thoughts. Bringing these to a place of inner acceptance and friendship is required for a successful union.

How much more powerful and helpful I would have been if only I had learned these lessons sooner.

I am putting the past behind and passing along what I am learning. By marrying my art and science, I am accepting and showing my humanness. My dream is to excite and inspire all nurses to acknowledge theirs.

L. B.

Meeting

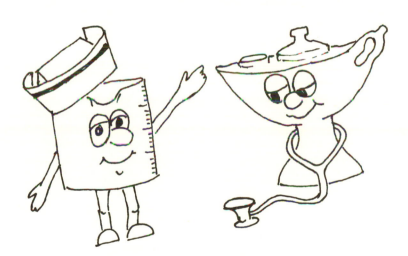

Dear Florence,

I met the one — and I want to run.
help oh help
I am fleeing this scene
for I know what it means
I will change and I am screaming out — NO!
Science and I can't possibly mate.
oh gosh it's too late
this part I hate.
I must open and let my true self escape.
Florence can't you see
I just want to flee.
oh why me?
the union is ripe
to let go of gripes
and grow with delight
taming and claiming
no more silly gaming
Florence, will you help me please hide
I cannot abide
yet I can and I will
I am drawn even still
for I see such a reflection of good
yes I should
stay the course
devoid of remorse
forgiveness will rule
no more hiding, it's cruel
Florence — today is the day
to show me the way
I will stay and be brave

not master or slave
I will learn to be friends
it is not my end
but a beginning of adventure
and gains for us all
I'll stand tall
and not flee
thank you, Florence
you'll agree
this pair could lead the world from its plight
I will take such delight
thanks for the advice
you always think twice
before sharing with me what to do
funny, I imagine all this
when I haven't even heard back from you.

With no regrets,
Art

Dear Florence,

HELP!
I was minding my own business when I bumped into Art, and oh my, I can't stop thinking of the creativity of it all.
My beakers sit empty as I contemplate the possible conflagration of our souls — what would this mean for my research and theories?

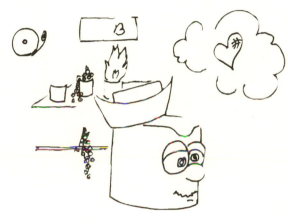

I feel as if Art would take over and yet intuitively (and I can't believe I am saying that) I know this joining would be great for each of us. As a team we would be unstoppable, but Florence I must hide for I cannot let out my feelings. I cannot let go of the position I hold.
FLORENCE , HELP
I am not ready for this alliance. I am certain there is better out there, And yet when I see Art, I see the missing link of the chain for meaningful success — I see the world.
Oh Florence, what should I do?
With jittery nerves,
Science

Dear Children, my reply to you both,

Art and Science, I hear your pleas.
I admire your courage to share your fearfulness.
You can and will summon this same bravery to move forward
with your friendship.
Slow and steady growth is all that is required.
Yes, I encourage slow and steady evolution with a strong belief
in the results, while enjoying, accepting and appreciating the
process.
This path is certain to lead to a deeper discovery of your
individual selves. You are miraculous beings.
Congratulations on the ongoing exposure of your leader within.
I encourage your individualism and know this will bring you to
a heightened approval of yourselves, where an elegant trusting
alliance awaits.
I foresee great and powerful outcomes for the future of nursing.

In anticipation of your further correspondence,
Florence

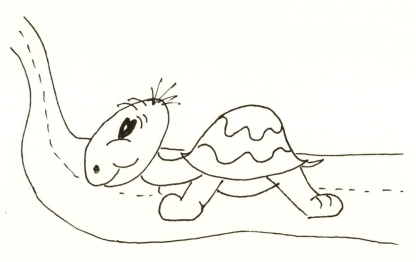

Identity Crisis

Example is not the main thing in influencing others,
it is the only thing.
Albert Schweitzer

What is nursing? Do you believe that we are definitely more than a list of tasks? Have we lost the art of nursing? Where has science been fitting in? Is nursing on a downward spiral, or can art and science come together to ensure its survival?

I used to believe that we all had the same vision and ideals. This isn't true. Human complexities make it difficult for nurses to explain who they are to others and to themselves.

Patients don't usually concern themselves with my quantity of credentials and certifications. An expectation that I am capable comes with my RN title. Whether I am kind, abrupt, hurried or harried, my education-based ability to provide for their needs remains the same. I think that patients are 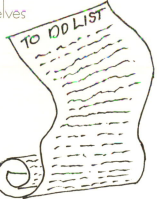 more concerned with how they feel around me, and how I communicate and posture my knowledge. My ability to assist them with their total needs depends on my experiential wisdom.

The creation of a nurse therefore encompasses both the knowledge and the education. To compromise either one is doing a disservice to our profession. Choosing to practice the science without the art or vice versa will hasten the demise of nursing, as we know it.

In the past, I allowed science to choose the path and pace of my practice. When I focused on doing only the procedures and tasks, my nursing care became clouded with the importance of outcomes.

Although I am proud of my science skills, my enjoyable memories come from moments spent touching patients.

I have realized that nursing is more about emotional and physical touch. Listening to the patient, teaching them, laughing with them and verifying my gut instincts are the experiences that hone my knowledge.

With all of the scientific advancements and technical approaches in health care, patients often lose their human place in the system.

Only when genius is married to science, can the biggest results be produced.

Herbert Spenser (1820 – 1903)

A loss of humaneness has created a sense of hopelessness, not just in patients, but also in nurses. I believe all of us are players in someone else's game, being tossed about on a whim. I've made a conscious decision not to lose track of how I practice my nursing as the game plays out above my head. I work hard practicing the art and science of my profession, to keep patients as the game's human focus. I do not always have control over the whens or the whats, but I do have control over the hows. My nursing care is not helpless or hopeless.

Several months ago, I entered the emergency department to a commotion and noise level that signaled a crisis. Two patients were in deep trouble, and staff were running to cope with these life-threatening events. The tension was thick.

Above all of this, I heard a loud banging and screaming coming from the private room often used for psychiatric patients. As I put down my briefcase, I heard an exasperated-sounding nurse ask the doctor, who was running toward one of the critical patients, for some sedation for the 'old lady' in room six. The young doctor hesitated, then

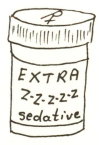

EXTRA
Z-Z-Z-Z-Z
sedative

shouted an order back over his shoulder.

The look on his face made me believe this was not a treatment plan he would normally follow. I offered to spend some time with the lady rather than just leap to sedation.

"You just got here. You don't know what we've been putting up with."

"I have some time. You go ahead and deal with the other patients."

Upon entering Room Six, I found Mrs. B. successfully out of the confines of the side-railed, elevated stretcher.

She was attempting to pee in the garbage can. I quickly retrieved the commode chair.

I spent the next hour quietly sitting and talking with this lady. Mrs. B. eventually told me what had happened. At her home, she awoke and stood up to go to the bathroom. She became dizzy and disorientated then pushed her 'lifeline' button as she had been taught.

Sobbing, she told me that when the paramedics arrived she couldn't remember why she'd got out of bed, and she became increasingly agitated trying to tell them what was wrong. The medics started an intravenous, sedated her and hustled her into the chaotic emergency room.

The medical service providers, paramedics and emergency

room nurses had frightened her into a state of panic when she was treated as confused and combative.

They placed in a dark, private room with the door shut to keep her screams from disturbing others. She had asked to use the washroom and was ignored.

Nobody had thought about or investigated why she might be agitated.

No one had listened to her.

As we talked, she became less frightened and asked to go home. I informed the doctor that the patient had not required any further sedation. He was pleased and thankful that someone had found another way to help this patient. The transition team nurse was called to assess if she required an increase in home care assistance. Mrs. B. was eventually released back to her own bed at the lodge.

I was disappointed in the initial response to this patient's plight. What might have transpired if I had not just happened into the department?

Sadly, I remembered all the times I also had not listened, and had simply done the tasks. I had forgotten that I have choices that allow a meshing of the science and the art.

The world is round and the place which may seem like the end, may also be only the beginning.

Ivy Baker Priest

Dear Flo,

I have this mirror in front of which I have been standing
for far too long, saying, "Mirror, mirror on the wall, who
is the fairest one of all?"
Is it me? Am I the fairest? Or is it Science?
I need to know.

Reflectively yours,
Art

Oh Dear Art,

Mirrors are not for checking who be the fairest one of all.
Mirrors are for the understanding and acceptance of
oneself as a wondrous creation. Then, by standing in
front of Science, you will reflect worthiness, as Science
will do this for you. Seeing the good and the strong shall
allow both of you to reach excellence.
Reflect to the deeper goodness of another and it will be
evident.
Ah, the power of the looking glass.

Yours,
Flo

Friendship

When someone tells you the truth, lets you think
for yourself, experience your own emotions, s/he is
treating you as a true equal. As a friend.
                                        Whitney Otto

Bringing together the art and science within me, and
making peace with each of them, is my goal. Examination
of the two parts needs to happen before any sort of lasting
friendship is formed.

My art — what does it look like? And my science —
what does it look like?

Science is the easier of the two for me to define. It is the
why and what side: the tasks, the outcomes and the black and
white. The art side of me is the who and how I provide the
science.

The who, is discovering my real self. Previously I did not
understand my art side, as I had not clearly defined myself.
This confusion affected how I provided care. Until I uncover
all of my humanness, I cannot completely balance the who
and the how. Art is the part of nursing that is
unique to each of us.

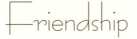

Working in emergency nursing immersed
me in the science. I was on a treadmill
that unknown sources had turned

up the speed on. I ran from task to task, spending little or no time thinking about how I was doing the procedures. At the end of the day I was exhausted, angry and unfulfilled. Something was missing.

I had compromised how and when I was performing the nursing tasks. As a result, my anger was building, and I directed it at the science of the nursing world. Today, however, knowing that nursing is not all art or all science lessens my dissatisfaction. And, I also know that when I attack those on the outside, I attack that part of myself.

Marrying my skills to create a stronger person is rewarding for me, as well as those I care for.

How do I form this lasting friendship?

As I am exploring the depths of my inner self, I discover why I react in certain ways. This awareness allows me to be more accepting and less critical of my behavior. In turn, it allows me to be less critical and more accepting of the behavior of others.

As in any friendship, the power of the two is stronger than each individual. It takes time to get to know one another. I may have lived in this body for close to half a century, but I still have not yet explored or learned all of whom I am. As I strike a healthy balance with my art and science, I am practicing the artistic science[1] of nursing.

I am now presenting to the world a healthier human nurse.

Friendship is the comfort, the unexpressible comfort of feeling safe with a person, having neither to weigh thoughts nor measure words, but pouring all right out just as they are, chaff and grain together, certain that a faithful friendly hand will take and sift them, keep what is worth keeping and with a breath of kindness blow the rest away.

Unknown

I've learned more about friendship over the past few years than I have all my life.

Why did it take so long?

I was unaware of, and scared to uncover, the truth.

Sleeping in my deep well of hopelessness was all I knew, until numerous events awakened me. Self awareness is showing me why I chose certain friends and why they chose me.

Previously, I gathered people around me for what I believed was their comfort and safety. I was all-giving, and felt so good having people need me. This was friendship.

When I would experience one of life's weakening moments and turn to these friends for support, I did not receive what I was looking for. Instead, I acquired criticisms of my actions, thoughts and feelings.

"Don't cry about it."
"You need to keep busy."
"Don't feel that way."
"I told you not to do that or say that or be that way."
"You're so angry, you need to see someone."
"What a terrible thing to think."

I would be devastated. I would apologize for bothering them and agree with their view of me. My inward chastising for being so weak, foolish and dumb was the next turn in the cycle, which kept going around and around. The belief that I was one huge walking mistake flourished within my self-fertilized environment.

These weren't friendships, were they?

Where was the unconditional acceptance, the supportive words, the belief in me?

Then, in my dark hole of despair, I experienced an incredibly humbling realization.

As a friend, I, too, was not giving unconditional acceptance, and not providing supportive words or belief. I was not being a true friend.

After many tears and much self-directed anger, I am forgiving myself. As I work on being my own best friend, my need to be needed is easing.

This self relationship contains numerous aspects — just being with myself is the biggest one. I take myself on dates. They are simple outings: walking through the art gallery or museum, driving to the mountains with a picnic lunch, test driving a new car, rising to new heights on the swings at the park, spending a whole day reading a fabulous fiction novel, or wandering the aisles at the fabric shop enjoying the colors and textures. Going to the library is my favorite routine date. I also buy myself flowers and place inspiring notes on my bathroom mirror. I am falling, and staying, in love with myself — becoming my own best friend.

Establishing respectful boundaries is another facet of my self friendship. I demolish old safety walls while standing firm to my limits and respectfully voicing them to others.

Asking for what I need is a difficult task, and I often become emotional. Because of people's replies, I believe they are judging me and do not hear what I am saying. I am working not to slap back, and to remain assertive and persistent in my asking in spite of my emotionality.

Working on a best friendship with myself is my life journey. It is beginning to take on a more natural rhythm. If I grow surly and restless, then I haven't been tending my self intimacy.

Becoming my own best friend is the blending of the art and science within, to become an artsi-scisi kind of person.

The greater my own best friendship, the better friend I can be to others.

Friendship is not doing for anyone else, but hearing them, accepting them, respecting them and, if they ask for help, aiding them in meeting their needs. I will be forever practicing this, for myself and others.

No person is your friend (or kin) who demands your silence, or denies your right to grow and be perceived as fully blossomed as you were intended.

Alice Walker

Blame, Shame and Claim

Self acceptance is the salve that soothes the wounds of shame.

Andrew P Morrison

After reading The Culture of Shame by Andrew P. Morrison M.D., I understand that guilt is a feeling of remorse due to an action, whereas shame is a feeling of unworthiness as a person. Shame is about who I am, deep in my core.

I think my family was confused about guilt and shame, because I grew up hearing, "You should be ashamed of yourself," or "Shame on you." It is no wonder I had problems believing in myself.

"What did you do that for?"
"In my day ..."
"You should do this ..."
"Go get that bell, you're not doing anything."
"You have to ..."

Certain phrases did not appear to be harmful until I examined how they made me feel. It was then that I realized that my inner rebellious child would rear up as I felt hurt and then become angry. These words made me believe that I

— 31 —

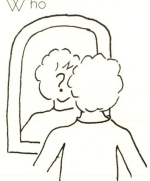

didn't measure up.

Negative talk, whether it comes from the outside or inside, was loud and full volume. Until I turned up the intensity of my positives, the negatives were drowning them out.

"Don't be so full of yourself."

How wrong these words are. If I am not full of myself, then whom am I full with? Everyone else, that's who!

I stood in front of my mirror, asking, "Who am I?" I had allowed other people to define me by their shaming.

Hear that you are clumsy or stupid or fat enough times, and it becomes a reality, a core belief.

And yet this message comes from the outside, other people's yardsticks.

Who told me I couldn't sing or draw or paint? An even better question: Why did I listen? Each time an opinion was given, I took it in and let it chip away at my self acceptance.

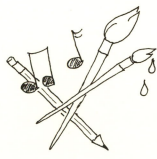

"They must be right, I'm just a loser and not worthy."

I allowed someone else's power to 'shame' me, and with each added criticism the belief buried deeper into my core.

Starting with positive self talk, I began to accept the woman I saw staring back from my mirror. I began to own my feelings, name them and look at whom and what I had been measuring myself against.

By taking ownership of my behaviors and choices, I may feel remorse for an action, but I certainly do not need to be ashamed of or atone for who I am!

I no longer carry the weight of shame on my shoulders. Only I can claim the blame, therefore no human will ever shame me!

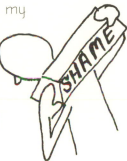

For me there is only one rule — simply self acceptance and respect. From these all things flow:

I will believe and trust myself.
I will ask for what I need.
I will feel my feelings.
I will accept my humanness.
I will show respect in words and deeds.

Working to accept myself also allows me to accept others. And because I am human, there will be failings. I am saddened to think how often I use words that blame and shame. Not accepting who I am prompts me to be judgmental of others.

Realizing that the actions of others are a reflection of my humanness, lessens my need to blame or judge. The saying, "What you do not like in others is what you do not like in yourself," is so true.

I do not have to approve of all the things that you do in order to like, be friends with or love you. Believing that the word 'shame' serves no purpose but to wound, I'm taking it out of my vocabulary. Not condemning or judging a person for their choices is a healthier reaction for me.

Showing those around me a different response from my old ways of judging, blaming and shaming has not been easy. But, when I say things like, "I trust that you will make the right choice for yourself" or "You are a creative problem-solver," it allows me to move from fearing our differences to celebrating them.

Me, myself and I, the three of us all one, vow that I will claim ownership and responsibility of the words I use and the things I do. Accepting that I can, and will, make mistakes allows me not to internalize them into core faults. I will learn from them and grow. I am not unworthy and I will not give others the privilege of defining my inner being. That is for the three of me to do.

Dear Flo,

Please Help Me! I don't know what to do.
When Art and I spend time together, we use 'cute' names for
each other, along with teasing and flirtatious behavior. Initially, I
found this to be fun and flattering, but now I find it upsetting.
It bothers me to be referred to as "the professor" or "my little
nerd."
I find myself losing pride in my intelligence, and I don't like this.
Yes, I, too, tease Art, with such words as "my little worry wart"
and "smothering mother."
Have I let things go on for too long to change them? Will things
move forward if I confront Art on this matter?
Am I just being too sensitive?

Tired of being teased,
Science

My Dear Science,

Teasing is a difficult subject to tackle because many people see
it as just good fun with no intended harm, while others feel it is
detrimental to their souls.
It's never too late to set boundaries, Science, and I believe it is up
to you to tell others when they have crossed your line.
If you do not respect your own limits, then you can hardly expect
anyone else to do the same. One must remain firm, not allowing
the sagging of standards. This courageous act is paramount for
the foundation of a healthy relationship.
I am certain Art desires a vibrant, lasting union and will respond
respectfully and honor your request.

Ever yours,
Flo

Boundaries

We need to find the courage to say NO to the things
and people that are not serving us if we want to
rediscover ourselves and live our lives with authenticity.
Barbara De Angelis

The boundaries of my art and science sides have been
tested in my practice settings.

Though the use of evidence-based
practice addresses the why and the
what of nursing, it is the how that I have
struggled to keep constant. Technology
has increased drastically in practice
settings since my graduation. Turnaround
time from admission is a field all its own, with bed utilization
teams and transition nurse liaison groups to help speed the re-
entry of patients to their homes and communities.

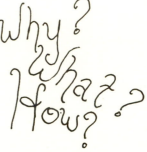

These new trends are impacting
the way I use my nursing time
and I know that I have
stretched my nursing care
boundaries.

Even as a seasoned
nurse, I allowed the pace of progress to affect the choices I
made. In fact, I chose to accept and stay in this speeded race.

Logically, I knew I could choose my own course and tempo, but I worried that I would not be accepted and respected if I did not keep the pace.

It was a Saturday, hectic as usual in our regional emergency department. I was working on the trauma and critical care side with a fresh young grad, 'keen, but green,' as the term goes. The shift was quickly becoming a nightmare and I was struggling to keep up with the needs of the patients in my care.

Five of the eight beds were occupied by patients with chest pain. Three of them were on nitroglycerin drips and should have been nursed much closer than I felt I was able to do.

Inwardly I was having the most interesting conversation with myself. "You can cope — no I can't — you've never asked for an augment before, why today? Why not? It's not fair to the patients, they need closer watching, they need time to ask questions and to get answers."

As a result of my self chat, I launched myself over to the charge nurse and laid out my request for more staff. She hesitated, hummed and hawed, then said, "No."

Wait a minute: "NO?!"

She mumbled something about proving herself and that she thought we could cope. I angrily walked away. Although I got through the day, my temper festered.

I tossed and turned that night, while going over and over the conversation. The next day, I confronted the charge nurse and told her that I was still angry about what had happened. Never again, I said, would I allow someone to tell me when I did or didn't need help.

As I walked away, she was apologizing and telling me her reasons. I turned and said, that I was as upset with myself as I was with her, because I had let the patients down.

"I wasn't prepared for your "no" response and I felt that you had challenged my intelligence. I became angry and then chose not to fight for the increased staffing. In the future (I said to her, and to myself really), if I ask for an augment and I am refused I will call the nursing director on call. I will stand up for the safety of the patients."

By stating my boundary, I had drawn my line in the sand.

Because I had 20-plus years of experience, I had not been prepared for my credibility to be questioned. Instead of sticking up for the patients, I went off into a corner to tend my bruised and wounded ego, draping it with anger. I had allowed my feelings to dictate patient care choices, and I learned a valuable lesson that weekend.

In my role as union president I was forever lamenting the rank and file members' lack of determination and willingness to defend their professional decisions regarding safe patient care.

What a smack up the side of my head I got when the shoe was on the other foot. It is still embarrassing that I could not walk the talk that day, but I came out of the incident with a stronger conviction to do better for the patients and myself next time.

Each of us learned the same science. However, we all practice the art of nursing in different ways, based on our inner truths and our view of ourselves and the world.

It was easier to look at my work life than it was my personal life, and within my work life it was simpler to examine my science rather than my art skills.

As I become more self aware, I cannot separate these behaviors. I am unable to perform my science skills without the art. Knowing that my personal life is interwoven with my work life, I can no longer leave myself at the door.

In the early 90s I sat on a joint union and management 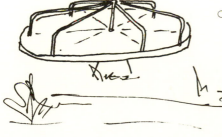 committee, created to develop a harassment policy. We went round and round about what was and wasn't harassment. The group concluded that it is an individual's decision to define when someone has crossed their boundary. It is their responsibility to stand up for their values.

Stating a boundary allows the other person an opportunity to honor it, and I believe this is the key to creating a respectful workplace.

I have a friend who hates being touched. For her it is that simple: do not touch me, definitely do not hug me. If someone tries, she immediately tells them never to touch her again. If after that her request is ignored, belittled or not respected, she would have grounds for saying it was harassment.

So if I knew about boundaries back then, why didn't I stand up for mine? Lack of self respect is my answer.

Today, I have stopped letting others define what I do and who I am. No matter what the 'norm' is, I do not have to play their way and my boundaries now reflect that choice.

A friend of mine was over the other evening and we were enjoying a drink along with food and conversation. We have known each other for more than 25 years and in that time we've shared a lot of sexist and crude jokes. He made a teasing suggestive statement and I did not respond. He looked at me funny and snorted, "You've not gone all prudish now — have you?"

I told him that I was being more respectful of myself, so I was no longer interested in that kind of teasing or joking.

Honoring my boundaries was also allowing me to increase my respect for men. Sneers and disbelief come my way when I state my new boundaries, but speaking up for myself feels great. It takes courage to stop my previous behaviors and I become stronger each time I defend my boundaries.

I love words and use them well, so well, that I have been known to cross the line of 'good taste.' Recently I crossed such a line with a fellow colleague. This young woman has grown from an awkward student to a strong and confident staff member over the past five years. I looked up from the papers I had been dealing with, saw her, smiled and said, "What are you doing on this unit?"

She replied that she was with the students. That's when I let fly my stinger: "They actually let YOU teach? Haha!"

Then I saw one of the students looking at us, and it hit me that I had just completely belittled this woman. I stopped mid-laugh and apologized for my comments, and told her how much I admired her taking on the challenge of instructing.

In the past I would never have thought about the repercussions of that 'joke.' After all, I was just teasing. I can't take back my disrespectful words, but I hope I lessened their impact by apologizing and speaking my truths.

Word puns and having fun with language does not need to cross the line into a tease/bully/harassment situation. As I become more self accepting, my ability to discern and define boundaries sharpens.

The minute you settle for less than you deserve, you get even less than you settled for.   Maureen Dowd

Respect

To free us from the expectations of others, to give us back to ourselves — there lies the great, singular power of self respect.

Joan Didion

There are layers to who I am, how I do things, and what I do. I am a woman and I am a nurse. Inside each of these are more layers, and further within the layers are my art and science.

There is beauty and art in everything. The beauty inside is left to the individual to unleash. My purpose is to uncover my art and let it be shown to the world. This is how I will show respect to myself and to others. The more self respect I have, the clearer I can see the beauty in everyone and everything. Showing respect is forgiving and allowing people to be who they are, and not thinking their behaviors are about me. As I allow myself my own choices, I allow them theirs.

Forgiving, believing, loving and trusting myself allows me to take responsibility for me. Doing these things is how I achieve self respect.

Most of this work is done in front of a full-length mirror. There I am standing naked in front of the mirror in my

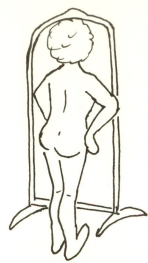

bedroom, with the lights on — believe me, that's a big step. Prior to this I looked in that mirror fleetingly, and with a critical view. Never did I look myself in the eyes and say anything. I was embarrassed at first, why? Because I thought I looked foolish — then I realized there was nobody else at home watching me. So why is it so embarrassing to look at or talk to myself?

Out of the closet came those old cliches about self indulgence, pride and all those other negatives regarding self love. I believe now, that those concerns about 'tooting' my horn did my self worth severe damage.

So I started my work at the mirror to befriend and respect the 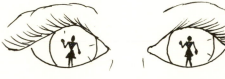 image I see. I look into my eyes and acknowledge the person, the soul inside that physical shell. As I do there is an improvement in my health and shape. The most interesting thing for me is the sense of calmness I feel as I acknowledge even the not-so-pretty parts of who I am — my humanness.

From this point I jump into trusting and believing. I tell myself daily that I deserve to be here and that I know what's best for me. I need to listen to my inner self, the positive voice. Ah ha — there is the next step, making sure there are way

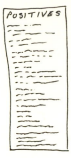

more positives than negatives coming from my inner voice.

At first, I wondered how I would alter or get rid of all my negative thoughts — images from the critical third eye stuck somewhere in my forehead. But I knew how to do this, my science side knew: practice, practice, practice. Say enough positives and soon you will believe.

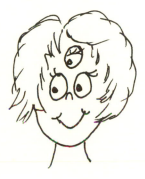

A pile of old crap came up while I was looking at my life, and I needed to get rid of it for good. I kept memories of past hurts and injustices cradled within me. What on earth I needed them for is beyond me. I am apologizing to myself for my past. I struggle with the face-to-face forgiveness of others, so I am writing down my pardons. By putting them on paper, I can vacuum them out of my closet.

This is the next step: I am taking responsibility for my part in my past, and no longer believing that others are responsible, or to blame, for my life circumstances.

In order to give nursing care without judgment, I will work toward self respect. I will be respectful of myself first, believe and trust myself, then I will be able to show the patients respect with my words and actions. Connecting the dots from self respect to respect for others and the resulting power of walking the talk is exciting, as it is so achievable, and so positive.

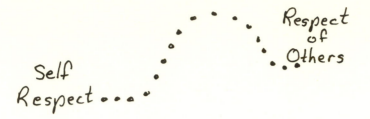

Always remember that you are absolutely unique. Just like everyone else.

Margaret Mead

Dear Flo,

Is humility all it's cracked up to be?
I am supposed to be proud of myself. By being proud of my
accomplishments, I gain self respect.
I know there is a difference between pride and ego — between
boasting over and over and being proud to speak of one's work.
To say I am a humble person is degrading, because
humble is defined as meek, unassuming, lowly and not proud.
I am not any of these things. I am worthy to be seen and heard.
Meek means I am subdued, domesticated and tame.
Oh my goodness, not me!
I am a wild, exciting spirit and plan to remain this way.
Societal systems want me to be meek and humble so they may
control me to maintain a status quo.
This is death, subservience and subsistence. This is not living life.
It is merely doing for the sake of doing, to be accepted within the
masses.
I do feel humbled by the sight of something bigger than myself:
the night full of stars, nature's power, the vast blue sky of the
prairies, an ocean's forever horizon and the height of sharp young
mountains.

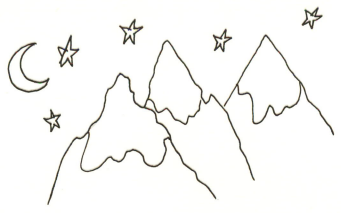

To be humbled by a person means I am less than them and I believe we are all created equal in the eyes of whichever divine spirit one sets his or her belief to.
Florence, it appears I have answered my own question.
No need to send this letter.

Forever yours,
Art

Nerditis and More

A peacock that rests on his feathers is just another turkey.

Dolly Parton

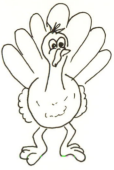

I confess I had nerditis.

Like the nice nurse syndrome, which I wrote about in our first book, nerditis is a disease that allowed me to feel needed, respected, loved and accepted.

I did not consciously contract these maladies. They were simply spelled out to me by society, gained by observing others and emulating their behaviors. I thought this was how, and what, I was supposed to do.

Man, I feel better getting that off my chest. No more hiding it.

As I wrote these past few sentences my mind was humming the song "I've Got Cabin Fever" from the movie Muppets' Treasure Island. Then I replaced my humming with these words: "I had nerditis. I had nerditis."

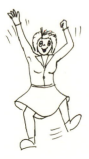

I see myself throwing my arms in the air to dance and celebrate this fact of my past. I can laugh and smile about it now.

"Oh! I had nerditis. I had nerditis."

This inflammatory infection became quite noticeable in the 1980s — it developed when I was working in the emergency department. It was actually smoldering when I worked in a small rural hospital for a year after training, but the flare-up happened in emerg.

Nerditis was a sign of the times: technology, new drugs, better methods and fancy machinery — advancement. I took numerous courses, obtaining BCLS and ACLS certificates, and then taught them.

I was proud to be a nerd — in fact I exalted in it. A nerd of the science of nursing.

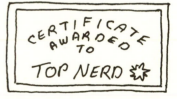

I strived to be the best teacher, regimented to rote in the world of algorithms and Annie dolls. To have a perfect strip of compressions and breaths was my quest and, once accomplished, I demanded others do the same.

One needed to be perfect and, at times, I believed I was. All this kept my ego fed with energy to use at work and in my life. What a life — I was a top nerd and it demanded all of me to maintain that status.

"Oh! I had nerditis. I had nerditis."

When testing physicians and nurses in ACLS, I was ruthless, passing only those who met my standard of perfection.

My bar was held so high it was nearly impossible to reach, let alone get over. Those arrythmias and their treatments came out of my mouth verbatim. I was a walking textbook and proud of it.

My electro cardiology knowledge began with Dale Dubin's, Basic Interpretation of EKGs, and I sailed on to study one of the masters, Leo Schamroth.

My PR intervals could stand up with the best of them. LBBBs and acute MIs — no problem. Heart blocks never fooled me. Wenckebachs were my world.

"Oh! I had nerditis. I had nerditis."

I read books on everything science in the world of emergency medicine. I wrote policies and procedures for the department, then configured and organized the formulas for the medication drips and infusions. I knew drug dosages with a snap of my fingers. I was an ace!

"Oh! I had nerditis. I had nerditis."

I had the nice nurse syndrome, too. It was a handmaidenly disease that I was certain would earn me Brownie points. The symptoms were in my words. "I don't mean to bother you." "Yes, Doctor. Right away." "I'm sorry. I'm sorry. I'm sorry."

"Here, let me help you." "What did I do to upset you?"

Crowd-pleasing was my aim and smothering mothering was my game — 24 hours a day.

Then I crashed and burned.

The nice nurse syndrome and nerditis were just too much for one 'perfect' nurse to handle. Bang — these diseases infiltrated my being and took control.

Who did I think I was — well, 'superwoman' of course!

There was no such person.

To be a good nurse, I believed I needed to be a combination of the nice nurse syndrome and nerditis. My equation looked like this: $N = N+N$

The overall self destruction from these inflictions was a rude but healthy awakening!

As I began healing, I let go of the desire to be perfect in both the art and science of nursing. After my wake-up call, I changed to a 0.4 position in emergency and began writing freelance feature articles for newspapers and magazines in all areas except health care.

Then along came PALS, TNCC, PICC line insertion training and speciality certification. Embracing science way too intimately in the past discouraged me from wanting to remain in bed with it. Nerditis was not welcome! I eased back on the science input into my life, taking none of the courses.

A calming of my nice nurse syndrome occurred as I came to understand its causes. I began by eliminating the "I'm sorrys" from my vocabulary and providing myself with more positive self talk.

Developing an interest in and love of myself as a whole lessened my need to be loved, accepted and approved of by others. I no longer wanted to be driven by perfection, and soon this interest in the 'whole' transferred to the patients in my care.

Who was that middle-aged woman under all those layers of dirt, past the alcoholism and beyond the poverty? What were her thoughts and feelings?

The patient with acquired immune deficiency syndrome became a human being with tremendous attributes and wisdom. He was a joy to discover and happily joined in as we nicknamed him Sir O, after Laurence Olivier.

The 90-year-old great grandmother, who folded facecloths for us while waiting for transport to return her to the nursing home, shared cranberry juice and memories with me as if we were old friends dining at the Ritz.

My perceptions of people had been previously clouded with the perfections of my nice nurse syndrome and nerditis. In doing this, I had judged them.

There was a critical link missing in the equation: $N = N + N$. It was the human factor.

In my haste and need for perfection I had missed humanness — mine and that of everyone else. As I uncover my humanness, I begin to heal. My nice nurse syndrome becomes art and nerditis becomes science. As these inflammations ease, a marriage of my art and science is possible. The equation now looks like this: $N = A + S + H$

A continued understanding of humanity is now my life-long adventure. Believing in and concentrating on this process allows the outcome to take care of itself.

Accepting and incorporating my humanness is the successful union of my art and science within. At this stage I more readily accept the humanness of others. This results in an artistic science approach to nursing.

The equation can then be further simplified: $N = AS$

$$Nursing = Artistic\ Science$$

As we approach a new millennium, at the end of a century of explosive growth in science and technology, it is fitting that leading members of the scientific community are starting to understand that science alone cannot fulfill humankind's needs: indeed, it has become a destructive force. We need a new kind of science that approaches the traditional knowledge of indigenous communities; the search for it has already begun.

David Suzuki

Dear Florence,

I am struggling with bad memories of past connections with partners. I am having nightmares about all the previous arguments, which erupted with name calling and back stabbing. Florence, how do I forget? How do I forgive?
When will I have a better sleep?

With baggy eyes,
Art

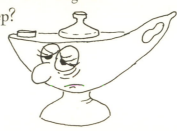

My Dear Art,

When I allow memories to carry such power over me, I lose all perspective as to who I am and where I am going. Yes, I fall prey to these moments of tears and anger based on my past, but I am letting go of the hold that I permit them to have over me.
Examine these memories and break them down into what they truly mean. As this dissection takes place, numerous answers are uncovered. These are life lessons. You will discover why you act in certain ways, who you truly are in your gender and which patterns repeat in your life.
My retrospectives are classrooms for self awareness and self healing. They are a fertile ground for growing my self respect. Realizing that all of us carry the same frailties, heightens my respect for others.
Embrace and thank your reminiscences. Forgive yourself for your humanness and move forward with your life.
Art, you are a wise being and I believe in your capabilities to move beyond the stronghold of your past. You are at a precious and celebrant time in your life's journey. Miracles of the future await. I know you have the courage for resolve. I believe in you.

In this memorable moment,
Flo

The Tradition of Permission

You can clutch the past so tightly to your chest that it leaves your arms too full to embrace the present.
Unknown

Dear Me,
I hereby give permission to you to be yourself. Yours truly,
Myself

I give me permission to be me. Permission to be all that I am. Permission to uncover my true self.

I like placing words into song tunes. "Permission — Permission" sung to the tune "Tradition," from Fiddler on the Roof.

Permission is defined as formal consent or authorization.

Why did I need formal consent to live my own life? Why did I need authorization to be me?

Because ... because ... because I believed I was not worthy to stand alone, to be independent from authority, to be a person — me — defined as self — moi.

I was labeled as Kathy, but directed on how to be her. It was the way the world was in the 60s and 70s and I grew to need this direction. I drank in tradition, allowing it to grow me strong and believing in its rule.

"Tradition — Tradition."

Over the past 25 years, I've felt odd — a slow rumbling inside that ached again and again. It spoke to me of freedom, a need for truths and a need to be me. I needed to express, define and live my dreams of who I could be, not who I should be. As a child I was born with this and then it was taken away.

I've awakened to the wonder of me. My truths are my guides.

Not following the acceptable fashion, I dress as I want and conduct myself as I wish. My dreams are now important and I am living them each day. I am becoming me, Kathy.

> You gain a self image from your past, not a self.
> Madeleine L'Engle

I own me therefore I give myself permission. I am the tradition.

"Permission — Permission."

Permission shall now and forever be mine to grant myself. I am equal to all others, therefore I shed the 'shoulds' of tradition — tradition giving myself permission — permission.

> ... as we let our own light shine, we unconsciously give others permission to do the same.
> Marianne Williamson

More Do Be Do Be Do

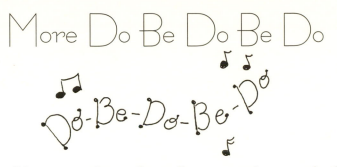

Do-Be-Do-Be-Do

We shall listen to the still small voice within us which
never yet has led any one of us astray.
Arthur Mee (1875–1943)

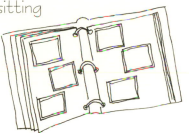

I used to think that 'being' meant sitting
quietly, taking time for myself and
recharging my inner fires. Now I
believe it is more active than that.
'Being' is relearning my self image,
those pictures seared into my brain from childhood.

Going back to the time when that image was scorched into
my beliefs allows me to examine that memory with the eyes of
an adult. Some of those past images are not accurate, and I
am removing them and replacing them with the truth.

Recently I attended a celebration weekend for my
hometown, and inevitably out came the yearbooks. Much
laughter followed as my classmates and I flowed back in
time. I was surprised to see that I appeared the same size
as most of the girls in those pictures. Even in the basketball
uniform shorts, I saw that I was no 'beached whale,' and yet

I remember feeling that way. I had spent all of my high school years feeling awkward and fat, yet there in full color was an average schoolgirl, not fat but not skinny, just one of the crowd. WOW. What a colossal waste of time all that worry was.

Now comes the work to remove that scar, and others like it. The 'being' is where my mirror work comes in. I look into the mirror and see, really see, not the image from the past but the reality of now. It is essential and rewarding work. Looking into my eyes and accepting the woman staring back is hard but possible.

I am accepted by, and safe with, my friends and I need to feel that way with myself. I want that 'blanketed with warmth' sensation that comes with the acceptance and trust of true friends. There is no end to doing my work in learning to 'be.'

Discovering how to be alone with myself, not filling my life with things or busy work, is 'being.' Dreaming my future while 'being' allows a vision to be set and I can then use my talents to step toward it. If I force my dream to happen, it will be stifled and changed. 'Being' is allowing my future to unfold on its own.

Faith is giving up control. I do not know exactly what my life is to look like or what I am meant to do. I believe that is not for me to know.

Be — the Verb

Life is about being, not doing.
                                   Elisabeth Kübler-Ross

I am a human being, not a human doing.

I realize now that the words 'human' and 'being' are put together for a reason. If we are human beings, then we must learn to be.

$$human + being = be$$

Be, a passive verb, turns active as we learn how. Doing was easy for me to master; 'being' is becoming easier.

In The Hopelessly Human Nurse: simple strategies for overhauling your lamp, I wrote about my start in the 'being' world. Initially, I forced myself to sit still and lie still, but my mind was racing with ideas for 'doing.'

When illness forced me to stay put, I read through a big box of old Mother Earth News magazines. I even made notes. This constant doing and planning while I was to be resting, along with the persistence of my critical negative inner voice, needed to be tamed so that I would just be. Calming my inner talk and doing nothing was not easy, because 'being' was ripe with fright — ripe with the unknown. I was scared of my truths — my frailties and weaknesses — the things that I thought I had no control over.

Choices began to appear while I was 'being.' Different angles for seeing things, and solving dilemmas, emerged.

My sense of helplessness and hopelessness continues to ease, the more I 'be' with myself. New habits form when I learn fresh pathways of behavior while shutting down old ones.

Although I have added 'being' to my 'to do' list, I often overlook it, quickly growing surly, tired and on edge.

"What is wrong with you?" I or others ask.

I re-evaluate my past few days, realizing that I have skipped my 'being' date. Developing a routine to 'be' takes time and effort. Understanding that its effectiveness relates directly to the repetitiveness of its usage allows me to appreciate its importance.

'Being,' these past few years, has become so much more than just sitting still. It is my time with me. Time for taming and eliminating my negative self talk and practicing self forgiveness. A quietness in which to ask my questions and clearly hear my answers. A period to devotedly practice a more positive approach to my self talk. 'Being' is training my inner voice to nurture, not criticize. 'Being' is full of a bounty of answers, love and encouragement.

Don't just do something, sit there.

Unknown

— 62 —

Often my 'being' time takes place within nature, as I feel relaxed, peaceful and at home there. Positive self talk is now a priority for me. Every morning before I rise and each evening prior to lights out, I admire who I am and where I am going. Voicing acceptance and approval of myself, over and over and over again, provides encouragement.

This is what has moved me along with my life.

Now, nothing is impossible and everything is probable. I take on projects I once believed that I was incapable of doing. My life is lived to its fullest, rich with meaning. I am becoming healthier and happier.

MT. EVEREST

Yes, I make mistakes, but I quickly forgive myself and move on.

To 'be' is to be with myself in positive, nurturing and loving ways. To 'be,' is to be my best friend.

I am a human being and I am supposed to 'be.' My 'being' will continue to evolve over time and so will I.

If you want to be happy, be.
Leo Tolstoy

Courtship

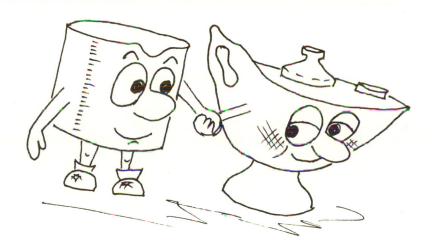

Mistakes: Not Right or Wrong

I love fools' experiments. I am always making them.
                                        Charles Darwin

Is there truly a right and wrong way? Yes, of course there is, because there are laws and rules that we must all follow.

So how do I handle my mistakes — my errors of judgment? Are they black and white, or a dull grey, stuck in the middle of right and wrong?

During my first job as a maternity nurse, I assessed a laboring woman to find that she was eight centimeters dilated. It was the night shift and I needed to call the doctor at home. This particular doctor was known for his temper, and if a nurse was wrong in her assessment when she dared to call, she would be berated and belittled. We all knew he only wanted to be notified at eight centimeters, no sooner, no later.

Being a new grad, the last thing I wanted to deal with was the wrath of a doctor. Confident of my assessment, I called him, then moved the lady into the case room.

I checked her again, my fingers searching,

searching. Oh No! I felt the blood drain from my face. Damn! I had made a mistake. The cervix was not dilated enough.

Why?

Who cares why, the doctor's going to be here any minute and boy is he going to be angry!

I hurried to the hallway to catch him before he changed into his scrubs. He was just rounding the corner to the change room and I spoke up. "Excuse me Doctor — I was mistaken in my assessment, she's only six centimeters dilated not eight."

He didn't say a word to me, turned on his heels and went back the way he had come. Whew! Well that went better than I had hoped for, but what had happened during my first assessment to make me believe she was eight centimeters?

After rehashing the earlier events, I came away knowing that I could probably make that same 'mistake' again. I had erred on the side of caution, but met the possibility of conflict head on. I did not run away or deny responsibility.

Reviewing the findings that influenced my decision making came early in my nursing career. I became a strong nurse, but I wasn't always gentle with myself when I made mistakes. Trying to understand why I made the choices I did led to self torment.

Today, sitting with my retrospectives allows me to search for a clearer understanding of what I am supposed to learn.

I reflect on why my mistakes happen and how I react to each situation. These inspections have helped me realize that my feelings of inferiority and insecurity cause me to be who I am, and how I act and react.

No one else can experience things exactly the same way I do. This knowledge of self, and of nursing, is gathered by my day-to-day being and doing, and makes me unique. Reflecting on my mistakes is an integral part of this knowledge. I learn from my mistakes and continue to do better. Self torment need not apply — only learning.

Dear Flo,

I find myself weighing and measuring everything Art says and does. I cannot stifle the judge inside of me.
Why am I so critical?

Here comes the judge,
Science

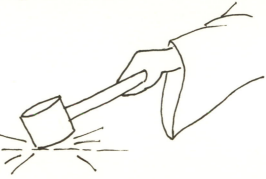

Dear Science,

You asked for my advice, so here it is.
Science, you have been measuring the results without all of the data. Your condemnation is not toward Art but yourself. Please explore the missing link — your humanness.
Once you start assessing your inner sanctions, the weighing and measuring will move from critical judgment to understanding.
The result of this examination will be a respectful acceptance of your choices as well as Art's.
Art will never be perfect until you are. Therein lies life's biggest test — gracefully permitting our imperfections.

Ever yours,
Flo

Mistakes Were Made For You and Me

Oh, I'm so inadequate — and I love myself!

Meg Ryan

oops!

"I made a mistake."

Four simple words, but oh so hard to say — at least for me they were. At one time, they were even harder for me to accept.

I grew up hating mistakes, shaming and blaming myself for them and covering up by way of excuses.

How could I possibly be so imperfect when perfection was my goal? I never attained it, but I sure tried, at times to the point of anger and exhaustion.

One thing I was perfect at was chastising myself for my imperfections — my stupidness.

"Kathy, can't you do anything right?"

"That was stupid of me."

"I hope no one else noticed. What would they think of me?"

"If I was only, could only . . ."

"I should have known better."

My voice was loud and clear.

What a messy jumble of nerves I was, even being scared of

my shadow, fearing it, too, might not be perfect or approved of.

To change my ways, I began by forgiving myself and accepting myself as nothing more than human. This is a continual task and it gets easier as I practice. I also choose to celebrate my mistakes now!

Congratulating myself for the wonderful learning experiences allows me to take responsibility for them. I laugh as I recognize, within each mistake, how human I really am.

No longer living up to the 'superwoman' ideal allows me to be hopelessly human. What a relief! Making mistakes does not make me a mistake.

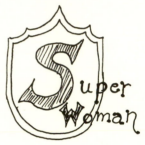

As mistakes became learning experiences, I began to see how sheltered my life was. I had become stagnant and dead, not trying new things or venturing forth.

If I don't make mistakes, I am not learning. I want to learn forever, so now I strive to make them. Well, not literally, but I take on new challenges. I risk.

A physician introduced me to the term 'blind faith.' Not being a religious person, it took me some time to put these words into perspective for my life. 'Blind faith' is believing in myself, and as I believe in myself I believe in others. Ensuring that all the i(s) are dotted and the t(s) crossed is no longer a driver for me. Well, not all the time! I simply believe in myself and work toward the outcome . . . never really knowing quite how to get there or even how to do the things along the way.

Do I make mistakes this way? Oh my goodness, yes!

Do I have fun and learn? Absolutely.

Am I a happier, healthier, calmer person? Yes!

Do things work out? Yes, and this continues to surprise and amaze me.

Faith is not belief without proof, it is surrender without reservation.

Unknown

'No', Again

The fact of the matter is that many children see . . . most of those who see are considered oddballs and every effort is made to correct them.

Carlos Casteneda

Why are youngsters reprimanded when they say "no?"

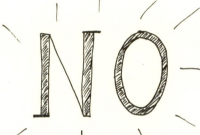

Children know what is right for them, yet are scolded for sticking up for themselves, because, of course, adults know better.

As a young girl, each time I was berated for saying "no," I grew more frightened to do so. "No" was hidden, to save my hide!

Negative replies to anyone above me were unacceptable! And in childhood everyone was above me.

Sadly, I left everyone up there when I became an adult.

Often inside my head I would be saying "no," yet out of my mouth came "yes." Doing this seemed right, while "no" felt wrong. Learning to say "no" has been hard. It's a tough word to spit out, especially with the often gracious ways people ask their flowery, sweet-laden requests.

Guarding my well being, and understanding what that truly means, moves me forward with my no-saying abilities.

With the summoning of inner strength, "no" comes out of hiding and using it becomes easier.

This single word affords me much needed self respect and this increased self respect allows my life dreams to be lived.

This communication change is not without stress, sadness and torment. As "no" comes from my mouth, I and others shake. I fight the fangs of my past beliefs, and the reactions of others.

"What did she say?

Who does she think she is, saying "no?"

What do you mean, "no?"

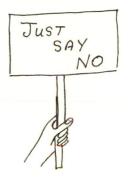

Kathy, what's wrong with you? You were always such an agreeable person. Why are you acting this way?"

Then came my ultimate test. (They always show up, especially when not wanted!)

I had enjoyed the challenges and demands of a bed utilization job for almost three years. Other dreams in life needed fulfilling and I now had the courage to set sail. Although my new adventure brought apprehension and unknown outcomes, I was eager to embark. I resigned my position, giving the required 30 days notice.

A few days before my final workday, my manager asked me to stay in the position longer. She had not yet replaced me and needed someone to continue doing the job.

I asked myself what was in my best interest, and
my reply was that I needed to leave the job on the originally
planned day.

I owed the facility nothing, but owed myself a great deal
more. Practicing increased love of myself had infused me with
the courage to respectfully stand up for my needs. I would
not allow those in authority to victimize me, causing me to act
from a subservient perspective. I was ready.

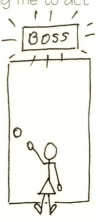

Boldly walking into my boss's office, I said,
"Regarding the request you made of me
yesterday, my answer is " "no"."

The earth shook violently below and inside of
me, while I stood firm. Man oh man, I felt like
gelatin on a rough sea.

The silence in those seconds after my "no"
was deafening.

I said nothing more and did not attempt to disturb the
dreadful stillness — a huge gain for me as I usually fill in
noiselessness with chatter, thinking that I am saving the other
person and myself.

I do not recall the exact words my manager said, but I
know there were very few. It was the shocked look on her face
and loud quietness that I will vividly remember forever.

Walking out of her office, I began to smile. I had just
slayed the demons that had stopped me from standing up for

myself. By putting my best interests first, I had maintained my self respect and my health.

As my office door shut, I inhaled a few deep breaths, because I had not dared breathe while delivering all of this! With a bigger smile, I pumped my fist high into the air and silently, yet with great enthusiasm and accomplishment, said, "YES."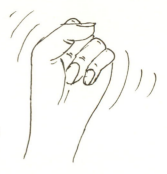

The inner conflict with my old beliefs was over and it had been 'my' personal war, not a battle with anyone else. My needs had been respected and I had believed in myself. Clearly and firmly stating my boundary, with no embellishments, justifications or snide sarcastic remarks, had also been respectful of my superior.

Energizing inner strength was gained that day, a tremendous courage to continue to say "no" for my betterment. I am worth it!

I say "no" when I want to say "no" and "yes" when I want to say "yes." Clear and healthy boundaries are set.

For the marriage of my art and science within, I am learning to say "no" to old parts of myself — past behaviors that kept me stuck on unhealthy paths.

Healing my nerditis began by saying "no" to further formal education. I had an instinctive sense this was not the way for me to go. Instead, independent reading, questioning and research enhances my wisdom.

To ease my nice nurse syndrome, firm "nos" were needed. Not doing for and saving everyone leaves them responsible for themselves and retains my energy.

My "nos" used to be delivered with add-ons: apologies, excuses or snarkiness. These are disrespectful to the person receiving the "no," as well to myself, because they assume there is an emotional and mental inability to handle the negative.

Two letters, one word, carries a great deal of power and needs no embellishment. For health, a firm, single "no" is enough.

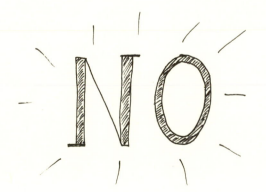

Dear Flo,

Just to let you know, we had a great time on our date to
the symphony. I learned so many things about music from
Science that I never knew before. Science spoke of a new music
appreciation when I shared my ideas.
It was all so very wonderful being together for the evening.
We each continue to hear music — maybe it's really just wedding
bells (ha ha) — but we hear it nonetheless.
At the moment it sounds a bit off-key, and this has us worried.
Science and I both know that a symphony's great music comes
from the sum of its parts, each section 'tooting its own horns' so
to speak — a blend of all that talent resonating to meet the needs
of those on the receiving end.
What would happen if the trumpet players   provided
their own as well as the French
horn parts of the score?
The trumpeters are masters
of their craft and could pull it
off with ease and finesse, but
somewhere down the road there
would be problems. Wouldn't
there?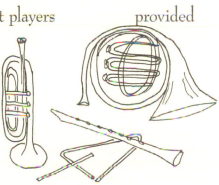
What would happen if a catastrophe occurred next and there was
no money to maintain the piccolo player? Hang on, though, one
of the trumpet players has offered to add this to his workload.
He said that someone has to do it, and he is perfectly capable of
taking on that small part.
Okay, saved again. No worries and the band plays on.
Then one of the percussionists refuses to 'ping' the triangle and
others in that section agree that none of them is going to touch
it.

The triangle is passed along to the trumpet section, which shows such flare and agility at juggling so many other parts that this simple 'ping' is of no consequence.

The trumpeters are exalted by their accomplishments and their energy abounds.

Stage set-up and knock-down for each musical event has become 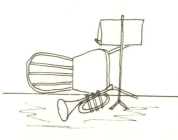 one of their tasks as well. No one else raised their hands to offer, so they felt obligated to rescue, and the band plays on and on.

This arrangement continues and the trumpeters are managing just fine.

They take sporadic sick days, yet no problems arise. The others in that section cope by doing double duty, and the band plays on and on and on.

The symphony's sound is excellent at the start, and although it develops the occasional hiccup, for the most part all the work gets done. This is all that is required to deliver an acceptable performance for the patrons. Then the flow of music wavers and an unsteadiness of the tunes surfaces. The trumpeters are sagging from the work. Their pleasantness disappears and is replaced by complaints and anger.

We can hear this symphony. We can hear the sour notes, the untuned instruments, and the frazzled spirits of every musician. The conductor bangs her baton, and the band plays on and on and on and on.

When will we stop hearing all this discord?

B flat,
Art

Anxious Moments — My Fear Factor

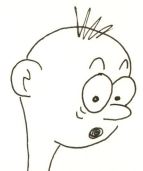

To give in to fear is to give away the right to live life on your terms.
Unknown

In the first book, I evaluated what fear was and separated what I thought to be 'true' fear from all those other things that stop us. This differentiation has moved me forward in overcoming these anxieties, of which I had a great number!

The fear of immediate impending death, which may happen before I can do or say anything, is 'true' fear.

I have been in that place a few times in my life and will never consciously place myself in a position like that again. Valuing myself as a worthy human being allows me the strength to communicate my truths and respectful boundaries. By doing so, I lessen the chances of near death experiences at the hands of others.

Fear is also defined as an unpleasant, often strong emotion caused by assumed danger.

What if...?
what if...?
what if...?

These are the 'what ifs,' and in the past I let them take over and run my life. Debilitating anxieties were ever-vigilant in my thoughts, and I chose to let them guide and control me.

What if I ran out of gas? What if I got lost?

What if I did it wrong and someone saw me?

What if I didn't act right, look right, behave right?

What if a 'bad man' was out there?

What if, oh my, what if?

'What ifs' were my whole world and I attempted to be prepared for anything and everything. 'Be prepared' was the Girl Guide motto I knew all too well.

If thoughts bring about reality, then of course I get what I expect. No wonder everything always happened to me. I was asking for it. I expected the worst to happen and it did.

Face the Fear and Do It Anyway, was the title of a book I read. I believed I was doing, this but each time I tried, I'd run and hide when I heard a criticism. Or worse, I would resort to my disgusting bullying tactics against the remarks of others.

I was a loser. My anxieties were just too powerful and I was just too weak.

Yet, time and time again, I mustered the courage to try to overcome what stopped me — sometimes my accomplishment was simply being out in public.

You see, I believed that I never acted 'right,' and that this was unacceptable to society — therefore I should not be out there. Was I even worthy of being on the sidewalk?

As a nurse, I found my uniform a safety net and the hospital building the same. Having a role to play allowed me to feel safe and accepted there.

Out in the real world, I did not feel safe. As a fat person, I have been tortured, tormented and judged my whole life. The 'sticks and stones' beat me down. It has been, and at times still is, a hard climb up to accept myself as worthy. Teasing and bullying were my life, and the words "if you can't beat them, join them" steered me to become a stronger bully and teaser in retaliation. I used the best arsenal I had — my words. They became cutting and I knew just how to deeply wound someone's soul.

I no longer needed to live in fear of being teased and bullied when I had become one of the best of both. While conquering the world, I grew to dislike myself and saw how others were turned off by my self- protective ways.

Today, I am letting down my guard and destroying my ammunition as I acknowledge, accept and exhibit my true value and worth. Yes, my fight or flight response can still be triggered by other people's words but I now have, and

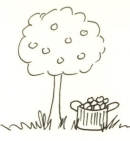

will continue to build, strong and clear boundaries.

I've read where sticks and stones are only thrown at fruit-bearing trees, and for me, I know that to be true now.

TV also instilled a great deal of fear in me. I watched human ugliness unfold each minute, each hour, each day. Between the homicidal dramas, round-the-clock ability to watch a war, and the exaggerated reality of the news, I imagined that horror and violence must be rampant in the world.

"The sky is falling. The sky is falling." Can you hear the words?

I stopped watching TV and began calming the irrational anxiety that every man around the next corner was a rapist and killer. Next, I canceled newspapers and turned off the radio news. The enormity of 'bad' in the world delivered to me to read and hear, over and over and over again, was shut off and thrown out.

As I allow less and less negativity into my life, I invite more and more goodness, positiveness and happiness. Yes, there is still bad behavior in the world, but there is way more good. If emphasis is placed on the good, it will prosper and the bad will wither.

I keep in mind that there is a difference between being brave and living my life, and being a stupid reckless buffoon.

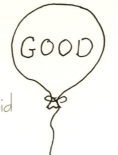

To laugh is to risk appearing the fool,
To weep is to risk being called sentimental.
To reach out to another is to risk involvement
To expose feelings is to risk showing your true self
To place your ideas and your dreams before the crowd is to
risk being called naive.
To love is to risk being not loved in return
To live is to risk dying
To try is to risk failure
But risks must be taken, because the greatest risk in life is
to risk nothing
The person who risks nothing, does nothing, has nothing,
is nothing, and becomes nothing
He may avoid suffering and sorrow but he simply cannot
learn, feel, change, grow or love
Chained by his certitude, he is a slave; he has forfeited his
freedom.
Only the person who risks is truly free.

                                        Janet Rand

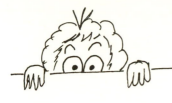

My anxieties are foolish worry about nothing. Fearful anxiety is rubbish and all in my mind. It is what I choose to make it.

Anxieties had controlled and driven my life. I have taken back the wheel and have a firm and forever grip on the helm. Criticisms from others are losing their power because their judgments are their fears, not mine.

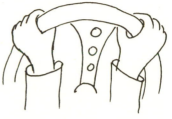

In the past five years, I've boldly moved ahead with my dreams and goals. I will strive for them, for they are who I am. I risk, for I now know no other way to live my life.

Everything worthwhile is a risk. To play it safe is to miss the point of the game.

Unknown

Fear of physical danger is not rare in nursing. I've been bitten, scratched, kicked in the face, spit on and slapped. There are also environmental dangers, where my safety may conflict with the expectations of the job. Static pours from the ambulance phone, obscuring the paramedic's message.

"You have a what? Repeat please!" Too late — they're in the garage already and I can tell by the flurry of activity that it is something unusual or life-threatening.

The gurney is being propelled into the department by two harried medics. "Knife wound to the chest — he's lost a lot of blood. I have my hand over the hole."

In less than ten minutes, we rush the patient to the operating room. The surgeon runs beside the stretcher with his finger in the hole of the guy's chest.

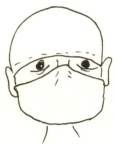

In the operating room, everyone is busy setting up for surgery. I was going to bow out and head back to my comfort zone in the emergency department when the surgeon asked, "Can you stay and help?"

"Sure," came my surprised response to this unusual request.

I stayed, doing whatever was asked of me while my co-worker from the ER was finishing her charting in the corner.

"Damn he's coding," and my head ripped around as the surgeon stepped back from the patient and demanded the internal paddles to defibrillate. There was much confusion, and then the words "I can't find them," reverberated like an echo in an empty drum.

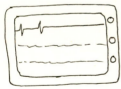

The surgeon looked at me and yelled, "Do it the other way."

He wasn't serious, was he? I mean, the man's chest was laid wide open and the rib spreaders looked like giant steel teeth. I couldn't even see any skin on the chest to put the paddles onto.

My anxiety level was rising and I feared for my safety. I was certain the surgeon wouldn't have directed me to do this if it might harm me. Yet, there I was, standing in blood, holding onto the electricity-producing paddles, attempting to get a flap of skin to cover the spreader teeth. As I prepared to deliver the charge I said a prayer. Looking up into the eyes of my fellow emergency room nurse, I saw fear. I pushed the buttons. "Clunk," the charge entered the man's chest. "Beep, beep, beep," the monitor responded with the return of his regulated heartbeat. I survived, he survived, and the memory lives on in my brain.

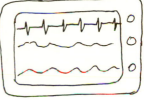

Should I have taken such a chance with my own life? If I had been electrocuted, there would have been two critical patients requiring attention.

Anxieties and fear will always be part of my being human. It is because of these feelings that I keep learning and reaching. The ability to stop and listen to those feelings before I decide to act is the key to lessening their negative impact on me.

I made my decision to defibrillate that day based on the tide of anxious emotions in the operating room. I endangered my life and did not trust and rely upon my common sense.

Trust and Reliance

If action flows from anxiety, the outcome is murky and disturbed. But if action moves with a swift joy and courage the world begins to resolve its difficulties and grow whole.

Bahauddin

As I gain self awareness, I am more consistent in trusting my art side, the instinctive intuitiveness that comes with knowledge from experience. Staying current with my science side through formal inservices and education provides me with a deep well of resources upon which I rely when making decisions. Both, together, decrease my anxieties, allowing me to choose healthier reactions.

I must admit that sometimes my gut reaction is to run, hide, and let someone else take over — anything to ease that panic feeling that comes when I do not know what to do. Over time, I've learned to trust and rely on myself, my knowledge and my skills. Owning up to my limitations and then sticking with the situation has greater dividends for the patients and for me.

My first nursing job was in a medium-sized rural facility. I was one of several new grads hired onto the maternity unit, and I remain awed at the wonderful acceptance and teaching the seasoned nurses bestowed upon me. It was because of their acceptance and support that I stood firm and did not run away from new procedures or situations. They reaffirmed for me that everything I did affected the patients.

One evening shift, I was in charge, and my friend, also a new grad, was my only co-worker. We had bundled the last delivered baby nicely into the nursery, and the mother was

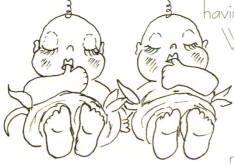 having a much-needed sleep. When I checked the newborn, I had a gut feeling something wasn't right. It made no sense, because the child was not displaying any change in his

color, respiration, temperature or heart rate. Still, something was not sitting right with me. My partner joined me as I proceeded to undress this wee one. A healthy baby lay in the next bassinet, and this gave me an idea. I placed the naked babies on the counter side by side, like specimens under glass. Even with my co-worker's added observations, we still could not nail down the what or the why that was making me worried — something was just off.

The next logical step was to notify the doctor, which I did. I found it hard to get him to believe in my gut reactions, but I managed to convince him to come and assess the baby. Within the hour the child was off to the city to see a specialist.

There were times during the phone conversation with the doctor that I almost wavered and agreed with him that I was just an inexperienced new nurse who did not know my head from my you-know-what! Instead of falling prey to my anxieties about looking stupid, I persevered, weathering his wrath and insults, and as a result won his respect. More importantly, I kept my own self respect. I had creatively used my science and my art together, solving a problem.

There is no running and hiding when I am responsible for a patient's care. There will always be procedures I haven't done, or equipment I am not familiar with, but ongoing education will ease my anxieties. The support and acceptance I receive from co-workers reinforces the trust and reliance on my gut instincts.

All these combined serve me well in my career.

Dear Florence,

I think that Art is chasing me. I'm feeling smothered. I need
my solitude — my space! This relationship needs to end. It is not
going to work. I am so confused.

Feeling like fleeing the scene,
Science

Dear Science,

I am going to be straight with you.
It is not Art who is chasing you. It is a lack of trust in yourself
that you are running from. The dreaded fear of intimacy.
Without these challenges, Science, there is no transformation.
A taking of space and solitude is a good
thing.
This 'being' time will allow you to
examine who you are and what you want.
It is a time to acquire self acceptance
and self trust.
Use this period to envision how you and Art will fit together, for
the betterment of each other and therefore the world.
Psychoanalyst Clarissa Pinkola Estés wrote that to love truly
takes a hero who can manage his own fear.
I believe in you, Science. I believe you are worthy of the best in
life and love. I believe that you can and will manage your own
fear.
Please let Art know what you are planing and why. You need to
respectfully voice your needs.

In the silence of solitude,
Flo

Feelings

We shall touch our emotion with reason and our reason will be touched with emotion.

Arthur Mee

I never seriously looked at my feelings and how they impacted my practice of nursing until my writings led me there. After all, I prided myself on being professional, not emotional, at work. This was perverse, because I couldn't shut off that part of me without dying inside. Perhaps, I was doing just that?

Efficient, knowledgeable and indispensable, doing the things expected, needed and rewarded — that was me. My hidden feelings weren't allowed to show themselves, and the more lost and silenced they were, the more angry I grew. This animosity turned itself against the system, the doctors, the managers, other staff and even the patients.

What was I supposed to do with all those feelings if I didn't experience them at work?

There was usually no one at home that I could safely vent to, but when there was I felt worse, not better. Never finding a way to stop feeling, I was ashamed of not measuring up to the assumed professional standard. I guessed I wasn't coping.

— 94 —

I channeled my feelings into actions when I joined the ranks of the union executive. Lobbying and fighting for improved work conditions was also my struggle for acceptance and approval. I became a crusader, the white horse rider, and the savior of the kingdom — anything to erase or control my feelings. It worked for a while ,until the horse bucked me off. I was so tired of the battle, and of my increasing anger.

As the hospital supervisor, I became more aware of the depth of negative effects caused by the widespread, stressful situations in the building. Deciding to let go of my anger and needing an outlet, I started to take toys to work. Child-like fun gave me, and the staff, a chance to laugh and release stress. What a lifesaver! I was positively affecting my health, along with the health of those around me, when my toys and I were playing in the halls.

Also, I no longer expected myself or others to just cope, or put it away for later. Now, I offered to cover if someone needed some time to deal with their grief or anger.

One evening, I was on a surgical unit when the charge nurse came around the corner, and in a hurried breath said, "I have something important to show you." Off I went, attempting to keep up with her, my mind leaping ahead to the possibility that one of the patients was in trouble. We entered a room and she pointed at the intravenous bag and sputtered, "Look, look, see."

I looked up at the bag and saw something flash inside it. The patient was calm and relaxed and smiling at me. My eyes darted back to the bag and I felt the blood drain from my face as it registered in my brain that the flash was a GOLD FISH.

This post-operative patient lying there, tubes in every orifice, had a goldfish in his IV bag! My hand automatically went to the roller clamp to shut it off. It was then that I realized I'd been had. The tubing wasn't connected to anything — it was wound up and hidden behind the pump.

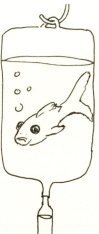

The charge nurse was cracking up, as was the patient. In fact, it had been the patient's idea. I was so relieved, and later I had tears running down my cheeks as I thought of the picture of shock and horror I'd given them. It was indeed a great joke.

That prank lasted the entire weekend, and many an
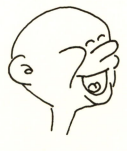
unsuspecting doctor and nurse were exposed to the phenomenon. The patient and his three roommates had a great time with it, and were up and out of the facility in record time.

I still smile as I think of how much paperwork I avoided because it was a joke. But more than that, it was rewarding to know that the staff felt comfortable enough to encourage this type of play.

Another of the fun things I've done was to provide each unit with an 'icky.' This slimy, slinky toy sticks to walls and ceilings and later falls down or slinks down end over end. The idea came to me from my friend, who'd purchased one for her son, and we had as much fun with it as he did.

The staff played and played with those sticky little creepy toys. They had a blast — I heard tales over the course of the week about the escapades of these toys, most of which had been given pet names. One of the units had made a stretcher from a tongue blade. They had bandaged the poor, now sticky-less creature and placed it on the stretcher. It was hooked up via a straw to intravenous resuscitation. No one was immune from the fun. Staff nurses delighted in the fact that the doctors enjoyed throwing the 'icky' around as much as they did.

Displaying my vulnerability allowed others to share that side of themselves. Allowing myself to feel my feelings resulted in an awareness of how I affected those around me. The more in touch with myself I became, the more others showed me their feelings — their humanness. The willingness to play, to be human, had a longer-reaching effect than I ever imagined.

On a recent shift I was deeply touched by the trust shown me by a staff member. This nurse is known as a tough cookie, not one given to any show of emotions. She asked to see me in private and then went on to describe a difficult problem she was having. Through her tears, she managed to express a total range of emotions, from anger to the sadness of a loss. She trusted that I would not do or say anything about her emotions, but that I would simply be there. It is a real privilege to be trusted in this way.

I know this is the way to create a friendship, not just with those we work and play with, but within ourselves. This is the way to bring the science part of me to accept the art side. I just need to sit and allow myself to feel.

THIS WAY →

Feelings are the connective tissue of friendship.
Joel D. Block

Dear Flo,

I am embarrassed to ask this question. It seems so very silly, but what is love? I get these 'feelings.' Is that love? And if so, how do I keep these feelings constantly alive?
Is love something that just happens, or does it grow over time? I am at a loss. I would like a definition so I can be certain that what I feel for Art is truly love.

With blushed cheeks,
Science

Dear Science,

Thank you for your excellent questions.
Love has been written about in poems and songs for centuries, and is continually and vividly portrayed in the media. Love carries many meanings.
As I review what are known as the four true feelings(mad, sad, glad and fear[2]), I see that love is not among them. With this in mind, maybe love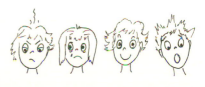
isn't a feeling. In the dictionary, the word love is described as both a verb and a noun.
To experience love I will uncover my true self from under the past 'shoulds,' 'shames,' 'blames,' 'harms' and 'beliefs.' This unlearning allows me to show limitless love to myself and others.
Providing love to myself, first and foremost, enables me to share it. I realize, now, that I can only give what I have.
 Unconditional love is an affection and caring for another simply for their being alive — a love of their humanness.
Please believe me, Science, this is possible.

Love is what we are truly made of. It is the happiness and energy that lives within each of us, often being covered over by other feelings.

Love liberates others to be their true selves and to shine their light from within. I strive to love all human beings, displaying an innate respect for them. We are all one and the same. We are all okay.

A love between two people is a respect for the other as an individual, with all the goods and evils of them allowed and accepted.

Love is seeing someone's total goodness and potential, and leading them gently back to themselves so they fully recognize and capitalize on it. The key word in that last sentence is gently.

I am very good at pointing out other people's faults. What I am honing is my skill to reveal to them their goodness and positives, over and over and over again.

As I accentuate my goodness and positives while accepting my negatives, I am better able to do this for others.

Is love a verb or a noun? Is it a feeling?

Are the senses that you are feeling, love? I will leave you to define this for yourself, Science.

What is love?

The well known 'Professor of Love,' Leo Buscaglia, said that if he was to define love, the only word large enough to encompass it all would be LIFE. He added, "Love is life — in all its aspects."

For me, love is internal. It is a gift I hold within and give to myself and then the world. Love within is my

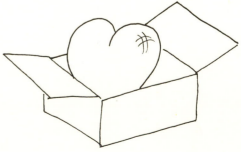

authenticity — my true self — and as I pull back the many layers of pretense, safety shields and roles played, my light is allowed to shine.

With respect and love,
Flo

Love is that enviable state that knows no envy or vanity, only empathy and a longing to be greater than oneself.

Joe McMahon

Crying Breeds Happiness

Your joy is your sorrow unmasked. And the selfsame well from which your laughter rises was oftentimes filled with your tears . . . The deeper that sorrow carves into your being, the more joy you can contain.

Kahlil Gibran

I have thought about crying, and cried, a great deal since I completed the Sad chapter of our first book. In it, I wrote about my newborn son being critically ill for several days after his birth, and how I was discouraged from crying by the one person I thought would encourage it — my older sister, who is a nurse. Nancy came to visit me in the hospital around the fourth or fifth day after my emergency C-section. I knew she was coming and had looked forward to 'letting go' with someone I felt I could trust to witness my pain and tears. Her support to grieve was what I'd hoped for.

I now realize that I had been unable to ask her for what I needed. I blamed her for not allowing my tears, yet I never directly said to her that this was what I wanted more than anything else. I did not know how to ask for help meeting my needs, nor did I feel worthy of having them met. I do now, and am exercising my self respect and abilities to ask for my needs, the best I can.

Asking someone to sit with me while I cry or to give me a show of affection and support during my tears is an undertaking I may struggle with for the remainder of my life. I am improving, as it becomes easier with practice. What I am learning is to ask for help with the understanding that some people may say no, and to be okay with that.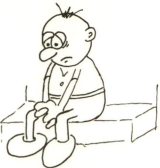

I believe people's own fears stop them from sitting with me when I cry. Given their fears, I cannot get angry with them. Having no expectation keeps the peace and allows me to choose wisely those around whom I release. I am learning to discern the people I can turn to, to help me with my needs.

Dr. William Frey, a biochemist and director of the Dry Eye and Tear Research Centre in Minnesota, has discovered that there is a chemical difference between tears produced from chopping onions and those brought about by emotions. The Centre has found that emotional tears have a high level of cortisol, one of the body's primary stress hormones. Crying is the easiest and fastest way to rid our body of emotional pain, so it becomes a healthy emitter of our wastes.

Tears are the safety valves of the heart when too
much pressure is laid upon it.
                                    Albert Richard Smith

Emotional tears, clearly, play a role as a
healer. I want that effluence out of my body,
not in, where it will manifest as a disease.
So cry I do while spent tissues pile up, and
I metaphorically toss all my crap into the garbage. It feels
wonderful.

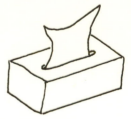

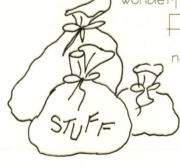

For me, crying is grieving, and I was
never really taught how to grieve.
Is there a procedure somewhere?
Protocol of dos and don'ts?
My tears usually flowed at times
other than the actual traumatic
event. I trained myself to shut down, and see now how the
'stiff upper lip' attitude was so very detrimental to me.
Judgments were cast my way at events where I should have
cried (note the word 'should') yet did not. And if I did cry, I
felt I was judged as well.

Guess what — I don't care any more. It is my life, and
I'll cry if, and when and where, I want to. As I do this, I
annihilate my inner demon, which criticized others for their
tears or lack of.

Now, I let the tears flow where they may, taking my

smudged glasses off to wipe my eyes. What a wonderful relief it is. When I look at those around me, the air is often uncomfortable, almost stifling, as if no one knows what to do or say. No one needs to do anything ... that's the beauty of it, just sit with me ... breathe with me. Join me, if you so desire.

Do I cry? Yes, of course I do. It is healthy. I cry for my losses and let them go. I no longer wait to cry ... I cry.

This being human is a guest house. Every morning a new arrival.

A joy, a depression, a meanness, some momentary awareness comes as an unexpected visitor. Welcome and entertain them all!

Even if they're a crowd of sorrows who violently sweep your house empty of its furniture. Still, treat each guest honorably. He may be clearing you out for some new delight.

Rumi

Simply Happy

Happiness hides in life's small details. If you're not looking, it becomes invisible.

Joyce Brothers

In December of 1979, I was working as a new RN in a 14-bed rural hospital. On the evening shift, a few days before Christmas, I decided to have a singsong and sharing night. The only patients present within the facility were three women and two men waiting for long term care placement, and a laboring woman whose contractions had stopped.

Dinners were served at 5 p.m., and once medications were given, clean up and treatments were done it was close to 7 p.m. 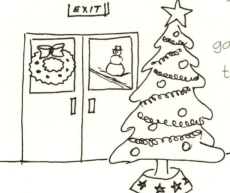 The nursing aide and I gathered the LTC patients, three of them in wheelchairs, around the decorated Christmas tree by the inner door of the front entrance. The seven of us formed a beautiful group. We sang carols and told stories of past Christmases, prairie winters and magical innocence. I watched as smiles appeared on the often somber faces. Laughter erupted, and eyes grew brighter and sparkled as the gathering came alive.

The laboring woman, whose room was right across from where we were gathered, rang her call bell shortly after we started. The aide went to check on her and came back, leaving the door wide open.

"She asked if the door could be left open so she could hear us."

Everyone savored hot chocolate and decorated cookies. Our circle celebration lasted about an hour. As I wheeled Mr. Gordon back to his room, he started crying. I stopped in the hall and crouched down by the chair's side, asking him what was wrong.

While the tears continued down his cheeks, he placed his hand over mine, which rested along the side of the chair.

"I can't remember the last time I saw that many people together," he said. "Or when I last sang. I'm crying because I'm happy."

He spoke of the tree, its lights and decorations. How he had enjoyed the hot chocolate and the candy cane that somehow appeared on his lap. Peppermint, as it turned out, was a favorite of his.

Mr. Gordon came alive for me that night and, I believe,

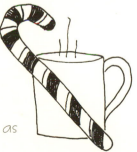

alive again for himself. Such simple things had caused him great joy and happiness.

In that hallway moment, I realized that this man rarely left his room. He was lifted out of bed and into a chair along the wall for meals, then back to bed. This was his whole day. Once a week he was whisked on a commode chair to a large tub room/bath area a couple doors down from his room. How long had he lived this way? Was it a year, maybe two?

Mr. Gordon spoke of his life more and more after that night. I enjoyed my times with him and worked to provide more opportunities for happiness in its simplest form. He began asking for them, as well.

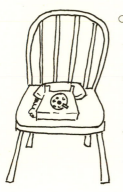

Spring arrived and, again on an evening shift when the only patients in the building were LTC ones, the aide and I took them outside. We headed down the inclined driveway that passed the front entrance of the facility and then along the street in front of the building. We left the door wide open, and I stretched the phone cord far into the entry, resting the phone on a chair. I could run back to answer it as needed. It was a warm evening, with the air full of lilac, apple blossoms and fresh-turned soil.

There were six of us out and about for the walk, two patients in wheelchairs and two on foot. Mr. Gordon, in his chair, was one of them. Despite our inability to travel very far from the building, we had a wonderful time. Well, I know I did as I watched all the smiling faces of those I was with.

Going down the ramp with the wheelchairs had been easy but coming back up proved to be impossible. The aide and I did not have the strength to push those in the wheelchairs back up the steep slope. What an adventure this was becoming!

There was no other entry that would allow us to get the patients back to their main-floor rooms. The aide and I helped the independent two inside, sitting them by the front door. She went back down the ramp to stay with those in their wheelchairs while I phoned the maintenance man to come and help.

Alex arrived, and as he and I were maneuvering one of the wheelchairs up the ramp, the RCMP stopped to find out what all the commotion was about.

While I was thinking, "Oh, my, I am going to get into big trouble," Mr. Gordon was chuckling!

It was an evening the whole town would remember.

Sharing my simple fun — simple delight — with others brings me great joy. This fills me with life. I am childlike and I love this quality of mine.

As I watched Mr. Gordon enjoy the remaining months of his life, I learned the power of pleasures' simplicity.

Happiness is when what you think, what you do and what you say are in harmony.

Mohandas K. Gandhi

Over the years of nursing in other facilities and other provinces, I lost touch with uncomplicated happiness in my personal life, and I saw it disappearing from my work life as well. I allowed the world's 'shoulds' to drown it out.

Gaining the insight that the key to my happiness is me, and finding it again, has involved an exhumation. I dig deep, opening myself to the multitude of choices — of how I see things, what I feel, when I speak and what I believe. Happiness is mine to choose.

The overhauling of my lamp is sending me along paths where I can and do uncover true delight in the simplest of things. Now, I concentrate on these.

The bigger picture of society, and what it thinks I should have or need for happiness, is no longer my definition of bliss. In many ways, it never was. I cannot buy it, earn it, marry it, eat it, drink it or smoke it. Others cannot give it to me, neither can they make me happy. I need to sit, listen, open up, look, hear and feel its pure essence within and around me.

Bringing simple happiness to the forefront of my life permits me to share it with others, magnifying its power to effect widespread joy.

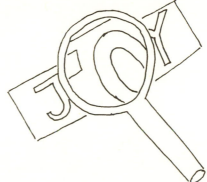

Savor the moments that are warm and special and giggly.
                                        Sammy Davis Jr.

Dear Flo,

Science and I had the most marvelous date last evening. We went for a long walk in the park and talked and talked. Oh, how we talked.

We discussed everything — past, present and future. I saw twinkling stars, yet I never looked skyward. Is this love?

We could see our breath in the crisp air. The mist from our talk enveloped us, adding to the magic.

That's not all — we found a teeter-totter. We came upon it at the end of the park, as if it were placed there just for us.

There we were, two grown-ups enjoying a child's ride. I never laughed so hard.

Guess what? While trying not to outweigh me, Science slid close to the handlebar and, for reasons unknown, let go of it. Science's legs were crossed at the ankles and, as if in slow motion, Science fell off the seat, or rather rolled under it. Science was hanging upside down for a short while before untangling the foothold and dropping to the ground.

At first I thought this antic was done to delight me.

Seeing the surprised look on Science's face, I realized this was not a planned escapade. I laughed even harder, tears coursing down my face and soon Science's laughter joined mine.

It was a delightful end to a marvelous evening.

Keep on teetering,
Art

Fun — An Innocent Turn of the Table

Locked in this dance is a secret language that tells the story of women's lives . . . their passions and their spirituality, their sacrifices, their joys, their intuitions, their emotional life drama.

Delilah

I am always dreaming up something fun and silly to talk about and/or attempt. People who know me are used to it — I think. Those who do not know me think I am crackers. This childlike humor gave me fun at work, providing a lighter atmosphere in which to ease the strain of an intensely demanding job.

A silly talk developed between myself and the ladies in the booking department of the hospital where I was the bed utilization nurse. It started with an innocent and playful remark about belly dancing. Once started, 'belly dancing' took on a life of its own and triggered numerous laughs for many months.

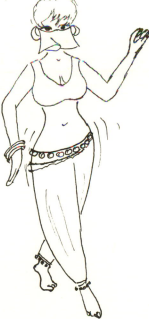

As the women and I discussed the gyration of our middle regions, we chose what color outfit each of us would prefer to wear. A couple of weeks later, one of the ladies confessed that she had actually taken belly dancing lessons years before and found it a healthy exercise. This began a discussion as to the express health benefits of belly dancing.

Over the next months, these ladies and I shared ongoing belly dancing information that we each gleaned from our own sources. A cutout newspaper ad for a belly dancer's performance at a local Greek restaurant showed up on the bulletin board in their office. Chat turned to what was really worn in the dancers' belly buttons as adornment. A ruby, of course, was the answer and this began a hunt for a ruby substitute that would suffice for us.

The next Saturday found a friend and I off to various shops in the city, looking for something suitable. Sadly, nothing perfect showed up, but many laughs came about that afternoon all thanks to the belly dancing fad.

At one point we were in a craft shop, and discovered those disc-like objects that are inserted into greeting cards to play tunes. My look of "oh no way am I going to wear one of those in my belly button and have it play Merry Little Christmas!" was all that was needed to move us to the next aisle.

Our laughter produced smiles on many faces and a truly

enjoyable day. Of course, the relaying of this expedition to the ladies back at the office was even more fun. I did take in small jewels to try out in our navels. Well, what a hoot. Amid a giggle parade, we tried them in on our various-size belly buttons. My biggest problem was that the jewel just wouldn't stay put . . . and on and on the story went.

Belly dancing talk turned up other places. My immediate boss told some of us about a great piece on a morning TV show, all about the healthy benefits of belly dancing. Oh my goodness, my office-mate and I howled, and tears formed as I let my boss in our fun. Our simple fun went on for months, with giggles galore and escapade plans for outfits, classes and ruby substitutes.

Many weeks into the belly dancing caper, a round table suddenly appeared in the office that I shared with the rural facilities' nursing director. Our space was fairly large, with a short distance of built-in counter along two walls serving as our desks. The addition of more table space was welcomed, but where had the table come from?

The mystery was quickly cleared up when Linda (my co-author) came to work for her evening supervisor shift. She'd found the table stored in another part of the hospital. It was clear that no one was using it, and she knew that we needed more

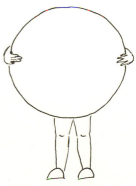

flat surface space.

She laughed and said that she 'got caught' while she was carrying the round table back to our office. One of the doctors had come along, while the table with human legs made its way down the corridor.

"Who is behind that moving table?"

"Um, um . . . me," Linda had said, passing by and flashing her best innocent smile.

"Didn't he offer to help?" I asked.

"Nope," she replied. "He just laughed."

Serendipity continued with the belly dancing tale, and our days passed chuckling at our antics, along with enjoying the new office table.

Several weeks later, I met up with the doctor Linda had run into that evening in the hallway. "I heard about the table escapade," I said.

He stopped, guiltily smiled and pulled me over into a small off- corridor. "How did you know?"

I smiled, and before I could explain, he blurted out, " Well it was the belly dancing."

"Belly dancing," I gasped. "What do you know about the belly dancing?"

"If you know about the table, then you know about the belly dancer. She ended up on the table I was sitting at, and put her scarf around me."

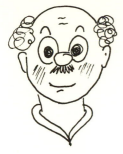 A blush graced his face.

At this point, I was howling and the doctor was looking more and more confused. I explained what I had meant about the table caper and then about the belly dancing. He laughed and laughed. "You mean I didn't have to confess after all ... about all of that?"

We each continued to laugh while holding our sides. You know the kind — those big belly laughs!

Dear Art,

I am blushing as I write this. I guess it is my
confession and I am ready to divulge . . . wait . . .
well . . . okay.
This is so hard to write.
Art, I am becoming a nudist.
Now, wait a minute. I need to explain myself and be clear with
you what this means. Possibly by being very clear, I, myself, will
be more aware of what this truly indicates.
I am growing more naked, yet I do not attend nudist camps or
naturist retreats . . . well, not yet, anyway.
I enjoy going unclad within my home and in nature.
There is something so totally freeing 'sans
clothing.' The air regenerates me as it reaches the
nooks and crannies of my entire epidermis.
And skinny dipping is divine! Soulfully sinful? Nah . . .
just soulful as far as I view it.
I believe beauty is more than skin deep and I am
stripping to uncover my beauty within — clothing is
optional. I'm laughing as I write this down.
Oh, Art, I feel so safe baring my soul within these
lines.

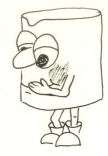

As I have been letting out who I really am underneath, I am
healing and accepting myself. I am a great deal healthier and
happier.
To truly unite with you Art, it is imperative that I strip down to
my bones and examine all of me. For our relationship to grow
and prosper I must expose all of myself, figuratively speaking.
As I accept myself, faults and all, I bare more to the world.
Many of the same feelings that I experience when I shed my outer
clothes arrive as I shed my inner coverings.

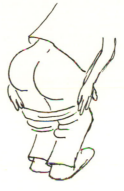

There is a release — a letting go — a freedom from which I gain energy, acceptance and self respect. My humanness shines.

Art, our marriage will be rich with truthful and open communication. I am prepared to continue baring all to maintain our joining.

I found this great quote from Dr. Suess: "Be who you are and say what you feel because people who mind ~ don't matter, and people who matter ~ don't mind."

I show who I am and say what I feel, for I am certain, Art, that you won't mind, as I am convinced you are a person who matters.

Forever em-bare-ass-ed,
Science

The Lake and I: A Metaphor of Truth and Courage

The opposite of courage in our society is not cowardice, it is conformity.

Dr. Rollo May
(1909-1994)

I approach the edge. It looks cold, yet inviting. One toe goes in, then another ... aieee! I was right. It does feel chilly, probably only 65 degrees Fahrenheit.

Maybe not today. I turn to go and my clear inner voice chides "chicken."

I turn back ... sigh . . . one foot then the other ... well, maybe it's not so bad.

Hmmmm .... okay ,okay it's chilly .... maybe, just maybe, 68 degrees . . . yes, but I can endure and will survive its iciness.

B-r-r-r!

I dip one arm in, then the other ... My oh My ... how refreshing!

I peer out over the water . . . so clear, so fresh . . . a mirror.

I downward smile, it smiles back. "See, not so bad," I say.

It looks like me! I smile again and again, and the lake keeps
smiling back. Now I know it is friendly. I sense its goodness.

The face is friendly and I pause to build trust. Trust with
whom? The lake or myself?

I ponder what I will feel like in there. Remember
the exhilaration from past experiences, I tell myself.
Excitement, quickly followed by calm, peace and relaxation.
Procrastination holds me firmly near the shore.

"It's just a lake," someone says. "You're not marrying it."

In my mind, I am. I am embracing it to build a friendship.

A partnership that will serve us   well. Yes, the
temperature is only 68 degrees. H_2O Two parts
hydrogen, one part oxygen with an   invitation for
serenity, guaranteed.

The lake has a familiar face. I will   be safe.

I ready myself. I steady myself. It is about trusting myself,
not `it.'

I look around ... to be sure ... no obvious dangers lurk . . .
no reason not to.

I slip out one arm, then the other.

I peek around . . . still safe,

then down one leg, then the other.

So far so good.

Atop one foot, then the other.

Past some toes, then all others.

There I stand — courageous soul.
Naked for all the world to see.
I run, hold my nose and leap. Down I look ... the face is
smiling back!
This is the 'real me.' I am as hopelessly human as you.
I have the courage to show it. I have the courage to let you
know it.
SPLASH............................

To be naked is to be oneself. To be naked is to be
without disguises.
John Berger (1918)

Engagement

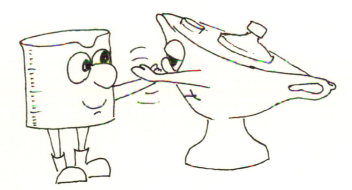

Congratulations Art and Science,
on your autumnal engagement.
Florence cordially invites you
both to tea at her residence.
She wishes to address with you a
matter of utmost importance regarding your upcoming union.
Please attend sharply at 2 pm.
September 4

Yours tr
Flo

Needs

I do my thing and you do your thing. I am not in this world to live up to your expectations, and you are not in this world to live up to mine. You are you, and I am I, and if by chance we find each other, it's beautiful.

Fritz Perls

I was doing a fair job at getting my needs met, but I was only addressing my base needs, not my emotional ones. Working hard to look after food, clothing and shelter, believing that the rest would work itself out, was what I thought was enough.

This was not true, and I find myself now wrestling with the aftermath of not looking after my inner self. I had been neglecting the one who used to dream, plan and hope. Somewhere, somehow, I had lost her — and the reason behind my life.

What did I want? And why did I not have it?

I would rant at everyone because I did not have what I needed. My lacking was outside of me, the fault of someone else.

Assuming that I had learned enough from my parents about how to get on in the world, I thought I knew how to deal with life's problems. I didn't know the half of it. Getting along in life means I have emotional needs. Getting along in life depends on me knowing what all of my needs are.

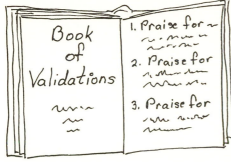

Self awareness is leading me to understand that self worth is a need. I am worthy, therefore I am okay to be alive.

Validations help form my feelings of self worth. They come as praises, either from me or from others. This is my base need, from which I move forward in my life.

I learned early how to get those 'feel good' responses from my family, school, and then work.

Having grown up in a large and noisy family, I looked hard for ways to get noticed and praised. Most of the acceptance came from doing tasks around the house, not for just being me. I wonder what difference it would have made in my life to be told, "I'm glad you are part of our family, I'm glad you're alive."

School came next, and any sort of praise from the teachers was for tasks like homework, tests, clean lockers and good behavior.

Acceptance from my friends and peers came (or in most cases did not come) from looks, style, guts and misbehavior. I was somewhat torn in the 'feel good about myself' areas at school, jumping back and forth between praises from teachers and acceptance from school chums. Finding a balance was difficult for me.

Work was all about doing more, and being the best became a way to earn praise and a sense of belonging. My inner voice would say things like, "They pay you to be here. They are not responsible to make you feel special or needed. You're patients appreciate what your doing for them; that should be enough."

Yet, I craved outside praise because I thought it was wrong and conceited to give myself credit. Other people's responses to me shaped my feelings about my place in this world.

Occasionally a staff member would say something that connected with my deep need for acceptance. "It's nice to see you. I'm glad you're here. I like working with you."

This praise of my person — my being — engaged me emotionally in the moment. I was completely there in body and soul, and my toils felt effortless. What a wonderful way to be at work, and I know I gave great care on those days.

If only others could feel what I felt inside when I heard those simple words of acceptance, not attached to a task. My heart

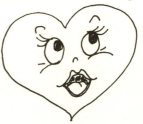

would sing and it felt full. I belonged just by being me! If I was able to recreate that feeling in myself, or others at will, what an improvement there would be in the workplace.

Not wanting to be needy or to depend on anyone else was a false interpretation on my part. My needs do not make me needy. They make me human. The truth is, these emotional connections need to be there for me to be at my best.

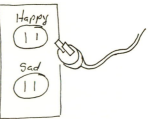

Correcting my imbalance means being gentle with myself and giving myself permission to have needs. I am learning how to fulfill those needs. Now I accept that it is okay when I need to know things, to study, and to use my brain, just as much as it is necessary that I learn how to be angry, to cry, and to feel. Thinking and feeling at the same time is my art and science working together. I need these qualities to be able to understand and care for others.

There are a few needs that I will ask for from friends and family. And it is with ongoing practice that I manage to fill most of my needs myself. Number one for me, is to tell myself that I am glad I am here and that I belong on this earth. I also need to know that I make good choices for myself. Now I look after my needs, believe in myself and celebrate by living my dreams.

Dear Flo,

I am struggling to rid myself of the nice nurse syndrome.
My identity came from this role and I was, and still am, praised
for my martyr behavior. Is this why I am unable to let go of it?
In the first hopelessly human™
nurse book, Dr. Stephen
Karpman's social game 'Drama
Triangle'[3] was described. I clearly saw
myself in its grasp.
Staying on that triangle as a Rescuer is
detrimental for me. This affects the type
of nurse I am as well as my relationships with others.
Florence, how do I care and not Rescue?

Persecutor   Rescuer

Victim

Signed,
Helpless in Alberta(a.k.a. Art)

Dear HiA,

I, too, struggled with the Rescuing role.
When I did tasks for people, which they were perfectly capable of
doing themselves, I was taking away their dignity. They lost their
worth as an independent human being.

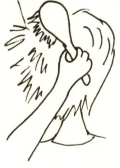

If I start brushing an elderly woman's hair after
she has fractured her arm, then I am dismissing
her adult abilities to care for herself.
If I take on this task, she begins to expect
it and when I stop she will often get angry.
I then become angry at her for not taking
responsibility for herself, yet it was I who

fostered her dependence in the first place.

My initial kindness was not really kindness. True kindness
is cheering her on with the task and celebrating her
accomplishments.

I need to understand that it doesn't matter that she has not
brushed it to my standards or that it took a very long time to get
it brushed or that she may choose not to brush it at all.

Being all about efficiency was my speciality, but now I believe
efficiency breeds ineffectiveness and disrespect for human life.
My actions kept patients dependent and this was a terrible
disservice.

I do not need to meet every
person's every need. This is an
energy-draining suicide.
Respecting others means that
I leave them responsible for
identifying and meeting their own
needs.

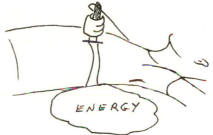

In my personal life, I also Rescued and at the same time felt like
a Victim when no one stepped forward to meet my needs or give
me recognition.

I can meet my physical, emotional, mental and spiritual needs. I
will risk asking others for help with them, knowing and accepting
that they may say no to my requests. I can and will accept their
decisions with no judgment.

 Art, this is how I continue to learn to care and not Rescue.

Ever yours,
Flo

Forgiveness

...forgiveness means letting go of the hope for a better past.

Unknown

I am learning to break my cycle of regret and self loathing through forgiveness and the creation of healthy self respect. Sharing these lessons with others is my goal.

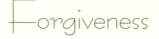

regret — forgivene-self respect — self loathing

I will rise from these feelings of sadness with a purpose.

Linda Bridge

These are the words that I said as I began to deal with forgiveness.

Forgiveness is both a need and a responsibility that no one else can fulfill for me. It is the true test of taking back control of my feelings and actions, and giving others back their own. I will no longer apologize for other people's choices. I do not have to take that on.

What I need to do is to forgive, in order to like myself.

How can I hate my mother, father, sister or brother, when they are part of me? If I hate them, then I hate myself because I am as flawed as they are. This is the viewpoint I started from and now have applied to my friends, lovers and myself.

Forgiving myself for actions that hurt is hard, and I

struggle with it. Saying the words "I forgive you" to myself is easy enough, but I tend to hug the hurt inward and not let go. Adding that hurt to the rest that I keep deep inside builds walls.

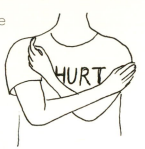

If I put myself in harm's way it is my fault when I get hurt. Similarly, if I don't forgive myself, it is my fault when the hurt doesn't go away. I deserve to feel better, therefore I work to forgive myself.

My choices about how I feel, think and act are made with the best of intentions. They have caused me reasons to ask for forgiveness, and will do so again.

Examining where my feelings come from allows me to understand why they are so powerful. I will own how I feel, and take responsibility for my reactions and actions. That way, there will be fewer occasions on which I need to ask forgiveness from others, or myself.

For instance, I struggled about which direction I should be going in my career. More education would mean increased opportunities, but I loved my role as a bedside nurse. I felt anger, then guilt over unmet scholarly expectations, and then shame, as if something was wrong with my being. "Why don't you have your degree? You mustn't take your profession very seriously if you're not trying to advance or be promoted?"

This inner talk implied to me: you're not smart enough, you're not good enough, you don't deserve to be here.

So I took those hurts and stored them inside. Now and then, they rise up and I lash out. I walk away feeling worse, having just attacked a part of myself.

This is the cycle I am working to stop by saying to myself that it is okay to like science (education), and it is okay to like art (knowledge). I am forgiving myself for past feelings of inferiority, and understanding that I can feel differently and act differently in the future. Forgiving will come easier as I become stronger and increase my self respect.

There are times when I have forgiven others for their actions, yet not carried on with the relationship. It takes energy to build and maintain trust and I chose to use mine elsewhere. Doing this is a healthier choice for me, and it is entirely appropriate.

Staying stuck in a place of not forgiving, however, causes barriers to be built that interfere with communication. Not forgiving keeps everyone living in the past, inhibiting human growth and acceptance. Not forgiving hurts generations.

Forgiveness is a new beginning, a starting point for understanding. Forgiveness is one of the healthiest things I've done for myself.

The day the child realizes that all adults are imperfect he becomes an adolescent, the day he forgives them, he becomes an adult, the day he forgives himself, he becomes wise.   Aiden Nowlan

Dear Art,

The word 'judge' has bothered me of late and I recently sought the advice of Florence regarding my turmoil.

Art, you accept me as I am and I accept you as you are.

We will falter at providing unconditional love, but the majority of the time our acceptance will ring true.

I am rambling and missing the point of what I want to say and ask.

Art, do we really need a judge for the ceremony?

I feel a judge will pass judgment and place a conditional environment upon us. I want, and hope that you want as well, a marriage that is open to our humanness.

There IS no right or wrong, there just is. Right?

I mean, correct?

Let's burn our measuring sticks, discarding the judge.

Art, I want to meet and grow with you in a non-judgmental setting.

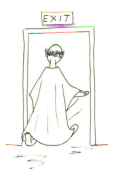

Out goes the judge,
Science

Dear Science,

You are courageous to write out your thoughts and request.

Yes, I will meet you in that nonjudgmental place.

Yes, I know we will falter at times and I am prepared to ask for forgiveness and also give it.

Our humanistic union will be aptly celebrated in the presence of the Universe. No judge required.

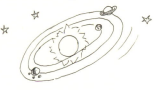

In anticipation of our rewarding future,
Art

Responsibility

The unique function of the nurse is to assist the individual (sick or well), in the performance of those activities contributing to health or its recovery (or to peaceful death) that he would perform unaided if he had the necessary strength, will, or knowledge. And to do this in such a way as to help him gain independence as rapidly as possible.

Virginia Henderson
American nursing pioneer

How wide are your shoulders? Mine carried the entire universe. I was singlehandedly accountable for my happiness, your happiness and world peace!

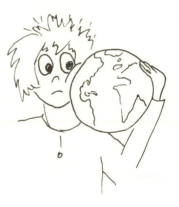

How many things was I presuming liability for?

Childhood issues, sibling squabbles and all my family's wrongs were my fault. I believed that to be an adult I needed to take these responsibilities on. Others wore their heavy cloaks of burden, therefore I hefted mine over my shoulders.

Somehow that turned into thinking that I was required to make others happy, wealthy and wise. Life was all about stepping up to the plate, and being counted on to do my duty. Oh, but I became so tired of the weight I was lugging around. I also admit, I took on enough responsibility to carry my entire nursing unit. I wasn't alone. Nurses before me had honed this skill.

Years ago, environmental responsibilities such as restocking equipment and keeping the rooms tidy belonged to nurses. Eventually, in most places, stocking clerks and housekeepers were given these tasks. Over time I found myself taking back the responsibility for the equipment, because when equipment was missing the patients were put at risk.

Ever try running a code with no suction? I would rant and rave at the staff. Lazy bunch, can't even look after the department. Whose job do they think it is anyway?

After speaking with management regarding these inconsistencies and receiving little encouragement of a positive outcome, I began every shift by assessing the patients, then checking, tiding and restocking the rooms.

Environmental responsibilities were not the only extra burden I adopted. I would play the go-between. Ah yes, that pig-in-the-middle game that always ends up with the pig in the mud hole.

"Pharmacy's on the phone — they need to speak to a nurse. Can I help you?" I said.

The drug the doctor ordered was too expensive and the head of pharmacy wasn't going to provide it. They wanted me to call the doctor and get another order. I tracked down the doctor, only to react with embarrassment to his questions, admitting that I had limited knowledge of why, or what substitute drug the pharmacy carried. In hindsight, I saw clearly that it needed to be the pharmacist who called the doctor directly.

Welcoming and hanging onto these tasks that were really meant for others was what I believed responsibility was. I confused being responsible with being in control. Taking on other people's tasks, and playing the middleman was controlling, not coordinating. I found myself in a mud puddle more often than not.

All this extra responsibility was stressful, and it was taking me away from the patients. I ignored some of the things that were my responsibility as a nurse as I wasted precious time on control issues. I neglected my true responsibilities of assisting patients with their mental, physical and emotional needs.

With regret, I admit that it was only recently that I realized what I had been doing. Now, I am of letting go these old behaviors. As I do this I'm like a pendulum swinging to extremes. Giving away some responsibility causes me to panic — no, no, take it back. I wildly sway back and forth.

Somewhere on that pendulum is the gentle rhythm of giving and taking. I need to find it in order to be a healthier person and provide healthier care to others.

I'm learning to smile and acknowledge, but not reach out to carry someone else's burdens. Using my art to practice my science centers me, in nursing and in my life. This gentler ride is freeing, infusing me with an almost giddy energy.

Dear Art,

I checked about a cake for the wedding.
The woman at the bakery advised me to
choose wisely. I could see nothing wrong
with any of them, and asked her why she gave
me such advice.

She explained that some cakes have gaping
craters that need to be in-filled with large amounts of icing in
order for them to look good. There is nothing noticeable on the
surface, but underneath the extra icing festers in the cavity. It
eventually sinks and, voila, more crater. More icing needs to be
applied to keep up appearances, because the previous Band-Aid
action only works for so long. Rotten icing remains deep within
the cake, maintaining, under the surface, an ugly wound.

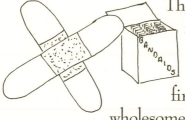

The bakery lady demonstrated how to
mend a cake with other cake bits using
time and patience. She shared a better
recipe to prevent abscesses in the
first place. It takes persistence to bake
wholesome cakes.

Her baking wisdom revealed a great deal to me about myself.
I would fill in my craters, making myself look good from the
outside. It was hard work to preserve this facade. At times the
messy old icing deep within would slip out when least expected. I
was embarrassed and ashamed of that ugliness.
I thought I was okay if I just looked good from the outside. Now
I see how unhealthy this belief was, because this is not being
authentic or showing my truths. All that cover-up. Who would
have thought I could learn so much from visiting the cake maker!
Not wanting my messy, ugly stuff rising up and spilling over, I
am mending my craters with authenticity before our union. I will

be true to myself and to you, Art.
This is a lifetime journey. Will you join me?

On wounded knee,
Science

Unlearn/Learn, Or: Who's in Control Anyway?

The first problem for all of us, men and women, is not to learn, but to unlearn.

Gloria Steinem

One of the hardest things for me to accept was my difficulty in controlling my emotional responses. I'm fairly intelligent, so why on earth could I not just 'grow up' and stop reacting like a teenager when someone hurt my feelings? Sometimes I got so angry I bawled, and I hated that.

I began examining what I was thinking when I responded in certain ways, or if I was thinking at all. Normally I am not prone to an outward show of emotion, because I had learned at an early age to contain those reactions. So I was surprised and concerned to discover that when I put my arms up over my head I would verbally snap at anyone within range — a physical action creating an emotional reaction. No being a human IV pole for me! It made no sense that I would get an overwhelming rush of restlessness and feel myself getting snarly. Why? What's wrong with me? Was I losing it? This lack of control scared me.

Warning: painting and wallpapering can cause outbursts.

As I told this to my mother, she started to laugh. "I think I know why," she said.

When I was two, I was on a Ferris wheel ride with her and my older sister. Just as the ride stopped with us at the top, I managed to slip out of the seat. Being a wiggly, active child, 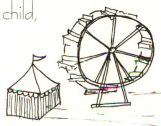 I slid over the edge of the car, luckily being caught by my mother's hands. I dangled there, kicking and screaming at the top of my lungs. Mom said I was so upset that it took all the strength she and my sister had to haul me back on board.

In the past I avoided situations that required my arms to be over my head. Now that I understand why those feelings of panic start, I can think them through, and build new responses; overriding my old fears.

I wish it was as easy to stand firm in the midst of my feelings as it is to simply write these words onto this paper. In fact, I was frustrated with my inability to change, until I picked up a book called The Primal Leader by D. Goleman Ph.D., Richard Boyatzis and Annie McKee.

There it was in black and white; an actual scientific reason why I was struggling with learning new emotional reactions.

The pathway where 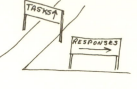 we imprint emotional responses is different from the pathway where we learn tasks or new concepts. The book went on to talk about this pathway being slower to respond to changes, as people must retrain their brains by creating entirely new instant reactions. Practicing new responses over and over is the only way to replace my old knee-jerk emotional ones.

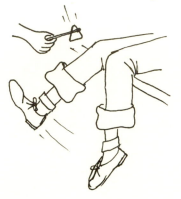

Flight or fight responses to fear and anger protect me from danger, but for reasons I am still learning about I have a distorted view of what danger is. My responses are triggered not always by true danger, but my perception of it.

According to research done by Dr. Joseph Dispenzia, D.C. (whose post-grad training included neurology, neurophysiology and brain function), our memory, once triggered, does not know the difference between our past and present reality. We react as we've always reacted, unconsciously doing as we've always done.

Wow, that makes me feel better. My reactions seemed out of place because my mind did not recognize that I wasn't in danger.

The good news is that, with practice, I can unlearn the old way, relearning and replacing it with a new response. It makes sense.

Now, I practice standing still and not responding right away. A big deep breath allows me to think about how I wish to react. Am I in true danger? Is there a reason for my fear?

Practicing conscious responses to old feelings is a time when being gentle and less critical of myself is essential. Creating new pathways to old triggers is going to take time.

It is a skill that helps me personally and professionally, as it helps me get out of my own way. This control is not the same as shutting off my feelings. It is becoming totally aware of them and choosing how and when to react.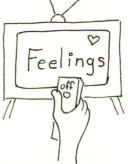

Entering into communications with an awareness of how I react allows me the capability of focusing on the here and now. As a nurse I can now concentrate on the patients' needs, not mine.

Dear Flo,

I'm sorry to bother you, but Science has me worried and confused. Science apologizes all the time, for everything. For goodness sake, someone bumped into Science yesterday and Science turned around and said, "I'm sorry." This behavior has left me wondering how will I ever know when Science is truly sorry?

Worried and confused,
Art

Dear Art,

My, my, my, it does seem that Science has fallen into a trap of fraudulent politeness.
It has happened to me. I was sorry for everything, never stopping to examine the truth of my thoughts and actions.
How could I be responsible for things that happen to other people?
I wasn't responsible, yet that was exactly how I felt when I apologized. I became burdened with the cares of the world, and so overwhelmed that I was unable to truly care for anyone, least of all myself.
The phrase "I'm sorry" is meant for times when we wish to show penitence for our sins and offenses.
Is it a sin to call a doctor for an order?
Does giving someone a needle classify as an offense?
Am I responsible when someone has to wait in the waiting room?
My use of "I'm sorry" had become automatic. After a time, I wasn't feeling anything when I said it and most of the time, those words were an untruth — a polite conversation filler meant to

appease. Their repetitive usage left me drained of energy.

I needed to alter something in my life in order to address how I was feeling. Therefore I decided to stop using "I'm sorry" unless I truly needed to apologize for my actions.

I stopped prefacing my requests with "I'm sorry to bother you" and let go of owning the world's problems, which further eased my "I'm sorry" usage.

It was awkward sitting through the silences that formed where the "I'm sorry's" had previously been. Mostly I carried on the conversation as if I had started with "I'm sorry."

I leapt right into the words I would have used anyway. Instead of "I'm sorry to bother you Doctor," I say, "Hello Stan," or if I need their attention I might use "Excuse me Mary."

It is not easy to change my habit of saying "I'm sorry," and I still find myself slipping into the old politeness trap on occasion. I smile at my lapse and understand that even if I falter and say the words "I'm sorry," I don't have to carry the burden or responsibility. I no longer squander my energy.

Back to your question about Science. I suggest that two of you have a heart-to-heart discussion about your concerns. Science might be unaware of how "I'm sorry" has become a knee-jerk or automatic response.

Art, let Science know you care and that you do not wish to waste time and energy doubting the sincerity or intent of your conversations.

Here is one more thing you can do, Art. You, too, can practice paying attention to your use of "I'm sorry."

As you become more judicious with its use your sincerity will increase. This respect for your well being reflects to those around you, and you will be a powerful role model for Science.

Ever yours,
Flo

Repetitive Communication

Communication leads to community, that is, to
understanding, intimacy and mutual valuing.
                                        Dr. Rollo May

I repeat myself, over and over and over again.
Others accuse me of it and I hear it myself, so
it must be true.

There are two ways in which I reiterate
things. First, by saying the same thing in several different
ways to others. I'm not sure if I do this to convince them of the
idea or to cement fully the concept in my brain . . . possibly
both. Second, I often repeat back to folks what they voice.
Especially if what they are saying is a direction or profound
statement.

Working in a fast-paced emergency department taught
me early to repeat all those verbal orders and, after a time,
to insist that they be written down prior to my carrying them
out.

My greatest learning moment, about this very thing,
occurred one evening shift. I was assigned to Room 2 A, B
and C, all monitored beds used regularly for patients with
chest pain, dizziness and shortness of breath complaints.

At the beginning of my shift, the three spots were full.
The middle-aged man in bed A had angina. He was pain-

free and stable, awaiting lab results and possible admission on telemetry to the observation unit.

Bed B was a young man with an allergic reaction to nuts. He had been treated with IV medications and was being observed. He, too, was stable.

Bed C was an older woman with dizziness and shortness of breath, who ended up having a very high blood sugar. An insulin drip and one-time dose was ordered. These instructions were given verbally to me by the physician while we stood at her bedside.

I merrily slipped out to the fridge, grabbing the vial of insulin that I needed. Waltzing past the drip formula book, I grabbed it along with the remainder of the equipment to mix the drip. I drew up two syringes of insulin, one for the bag and one for the patient. Then I had them checked by another nurse, stating to her the order I had received. I shot the IV dose into the 500ml bag of saline and we each signed the identification tag for the drip.

Passing behind the doctor while he was writing the orders on the chart, I returned to the lady's bedside. She already had an IV in place, so I checked its patency and to see if the correct solution was running, then gave her the one-time, IV dose and flushed the line. I piggybacked the insulin drip and placed it through the infuser, dialing in the ordered dosage.

I checked her vitals, asked if she needed anything, then headed out to the desk to chart.

As I began signing off the written orders, there it was . . . the insulin one-time dose had been ordered as a subcutaneous injection followed by the drip order and repeat blood sugar level in four hours.

S.C!

I was stunned, because I had assumed due to the level of her blood sugar that the dose would be given IV. I was certain that I'd heard the doctor give this order.

I went back to the patient and turned off the insulin drip.

Finding the doctor, who was down the hallway with another patient, I explained my error.

"Well, her sugar will certainly get better faster," he said. "Check her blood sugar via the lab in an hour and leave the drip off until then."

I sent the requisition for the repeat blood sugar and then filled out a medication error form.

Why did I start to repeat things? Because it leaves much less room for an error such as this one. This repetition is now ingrained in me from years of working in an area where life-threatening mistakes were all too possible.

Although I no longer work as an acute care nurse, I use my habit for another purpose within my communications. If I have not fully understood something that someone is saying, I will repeat back to them what I thought they said to check out my comprehension. Numerous times, people will use words which lead me to believe they mean one thing when in fact they mean something very different.

Time and time again, as I clarify what I hear, I gain a fuller understanding of what others want to convey. Prior to doing this, I would take away a whole different idea and be left muttering to myself about that person and what they had said. I am continually amazed at how conversations can be so riddled with misinterpretation, and that this is left to smolder and grow into huge problems.

Sometimes I will actually say the words, "I need to clarify this with you. When you said such and such, I understood it to be such and such."

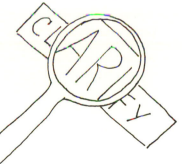

My repeating things for clarification brings me criticism. I don't care, because if my repetition allows me a clearer understanding, this will lead to healthier and happier relationships with others, professionally and personally.

I also ask others to repeat what they say, and often

find them changing words in the second verbalizing of their thoughts, giving a whole other meaning than what I had interpreted the first time around.

For me now, communication is no longer about speed or what I had thought was politeness, it is all about a true understanding of what others and I mean.

The simple transfer of my previous reiteration habit, into the everyday world, has allowed me to be clearer in my communications. As well, wordy repetitiveness aids my personal growth and change. When I repeat kind and positive assertions to myself, over and over and over again — when I repeat new responses to old emotions — my poisonous negative thoughts, words and actions abate.

Whether it's relearning a response to holding my arms over my head or learning to replace the "I'm sorrys," the verbal restatement process is my solution from within. It's an echoing answer to many life dilemmas.

This resonating repetitiveness of mine serves me well.

Recurring and recurring and recurring, again and again and again.

Dear Flo,

Help! I am at my wit's end. My need for Art is deep, yet I feel
unworthy. Yes, me, Science, who excels at numbers, research and
truth, feels inferior in the presence of Art.
Who am I to keep such company?
I watch as people celebrate Art's abilities to soothe and creatively
comfort those in need. I believed my academic path would make
me a superior nurse. I do not feel this way. Something is clearly
lacking and
I need your advice.
How can I compete with Art?

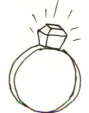

Diamond in the rough,
Science

Dear Diamond in the Rough,

I do not see your relationship as a competition.
Listen here, Science, it will do no one any favors, you feeling so
low about yourself. Be proud of your accomplishments. You are
admired and approved of.
Do not fear rejection and abandonment from Art. It is self
abandonment and rejection you need to be concerned with.
Please look into your mirror and make friends with the person
standing there. Once you have done that you can more easily join
with Art.
As you each uncover your inner gem and polish it to brightness,
your relationship will sparkle.
Each individual facet is required to practice nursing.

Ever yours,
Flo

Analytic Intuition or Intuitive Analysis

Organizational effectiveness does not lie in that narrow minded concept called rationality. It lies in the blend of clearheaded logic and powerful intuition.

Henry Mintzberg

I believe intuition is present within everyone, and I am confident that with practice our sixth sense can develop, becoming clearly defined within each of us.

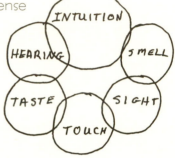

The dictionary describes intuition as the power or faculty of knowing things without conscious reasoning. That sounds like my inner voice, and in fact that is how I view intuition now.

As far back as I can remember, I've had a knowing. There were places and situations as a child that left me with a sense of uneasiness — at times, a fear of being there.

These were dismissed as silly childhood fears, yet I knew there was something more to it than that. Often, I learned the 'something more' later in life. Skeletons were moved out of closets and the stories behind them were shared with me.

I come from a lineage steeped with intuitive powers. My paternal grandmother was born in 1880 to a gypsy family in Britain. She never spoke with me of clairvoyance, yet I could feel a deep mystique about her.

My maternal grandparents were active in the Canadian spiritualism world of the early 1900s. They researched in Manitoba with Dr. John Hamilton, who was known for his work within this body of science. He collaborated with numerous world figures, one being Sir Arthur Conan Doyle. My maternal grandmother was a medium at seances held at his residence, 'Hamilton House,' which is now a fashionable boutique along a busy Winnipeg street.

Yes, I come from 'a past.' How could I not believe in intuition?

As a teenager, I began 'reading' cards. It was entertainment 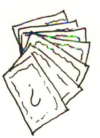 at parties. After a time this skill frightened me, because I was able to tell stories of others that were true. Being unable to explain how I did it unnerved me, so I stopped.

What started when I was 15 became a refining of my natural intuitive abilities. Slowly and steadily they developed, and I was able to visualize objects and events.

My roommate in nursing school residence once asked me to predict what mail would come for her the next day. I

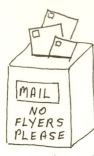

closed my eyes, visualizing the rows of mailboxes in the basement of our building, then I zoomed in on hers and peeked inside. I told her that there were two legal-size white envelopes and an envelope that was mauve in color with violets printed on the back flap.

I remember saying, "Sue, I can't figure this out, the stationery is yours." We both laughed. Then I said, "Wait, hang on, there is a package that won't fit in the box and the housemother will call you to let you know she has it at her desk."

The next day at noon, Sue rushed into our room waving envelopes in her hand.

"They're here," she said, showing me two white legal-size envelopes and, yes, a mauve one. Sue held it up and said, "It's from my grandmother and this is the stationery I gave her as a present a few years ago."

I was just as surprised as Sue about my ability to predict the mail. Then the call buzzer system beeped in the room and Sue answered it. One of the housemothers said, "There's a package for Sue at the desk, she can pick it up anytime. It wouldn't fit into the mailbox."

As Sue replied, "Thanks," then let go of the button, we both screamed.

All this again scared me and I again stopped tapping into

this intuitive power.

My first job as an RN was in a 14-bed rural facility. I worked the day shift with a 'charge' RN and usually an LPN. The evening and night shift I worked the majority of the time with a nurse's aide, infrequently with an LPN.

Intuition played a big role in how I cared for patients on my own. I'd have a sense that something just wasn't right and would check them again and yes! They were unconscious or had no blood pressure or had stopped breathing. I began relying on these premonitions and always acted on them.

A year and a half later I started working in a city emergency department and continued to hone my intuitive skills. At times, the department was a chaotic, crazy place, yet through all this mayhem, my intuition spoke to me. It often put me in a room at the moment of critical need. It sent me to speak with the doctor about a nagging concern regarding a patient, despite there being no outward sign to prove otherwise. More often than not, my hunch was correct.

My intuitiveness played a big role in my triaging abilities. That feeling would sway me to place a patient on a stretcher closer to the desk, or in a cardiac monitored bed, just because. And sure enough . . .

I have heard many stories of nurses' intuitiveness, as well as that of mothers. I believe intuitiveness is an art.

The only real valuable thing is intuition.
Albert Einstein

I am also a very analytical woman. I need all, and I mean all, the information before I will come to a conclusion. This need often stops me from moving forward with projects until I have gathered every piece of relevant information and answered all the questions — these being the why and how inquiries. This is clearly my science side.

What used to happen, more often than not, was that I chose one way or the other to react. I answered and moved based on intuition or analysis — art or science.

Occasionally the two came together and this is where my most competent and rewarding nursing arrived from. I wrote 'occasionally' in that last sentence, yet truly feel my art and science merged fairly often.

One of the most powerful events in my career, which signified to me a melding of my art and science, came on the night shift in a city emergency department.

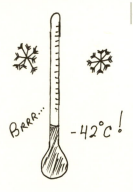

It was -42° Celsius outside with the wind and snow blowing. Two patients were 'sleeping over' to have repeat blood work done in the morning and there were no other patients in the department. This was an unusually quiet night.

BRRR... -42°c !

The public entrance was not manned after 11 p.m., but the door system set off a buzzer to alert us that someone had entered.

I was checking equipment in the resuscitation room, around the corner from the door, when the buzzer sounded. I headed out to check.

Three young men were half helping, half dragging another young fellow toward me. The patient did not appear to be drunk and I asked them what the problem was.

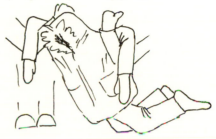

They explained they'd found their friend lying in his apartment, and he would not respond to them in any way. At first, they had thought he was playing a trick but it became apparent he was not.

"What's wrong with him? He seems 'dead,' yet breathing," said one of the friends.

The three helpers were visibly shaken by the state of this young man. They assisted me to hoist him onto a stretcher and I put the side rails up, asking them to give information to the other nurse.

I did seem dead. His eyes were blank and staring off into nothing. He would not focus on me or anything else remotely real.

Once on the stretcher he rolled to his left side, facing the

wall, and curled into a foetal
ball. I shut the door, leaving him
and me alone. Breathing, mine
much more audible than his, and
the sweep of the clock mechanism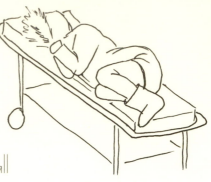
on the wall were all
I heard.
J would allow me to move his arms, so I
took his parka off. He did not assist me but
neither did he resist what I was doing. Once
the coat was off, J returned to his previous position, as if
there was a valley in the mattress that he just automatically
settled back into.

After taking his vital signs I covered him with a blanket
and asked him numerous assessment questions. Not a word
came out . . . just breathing.

As I left the room to chart my findings, I informed J of
what I was doing, where I was going and when I would return.
I left the door open and at the main desk filled in his chart
and wrote out my summary on the nursing note sheet. The
department remained as it had earlier, very quiet.

The doctor working in the hospital that night was busy in
ICU with two critical patients. One of my nursing colleagues
had paged him to advise him of this recent patient. The
doctor would come to examine him once the critical patients

had settled.

I could have just finished checking the equipment, leaving J resting in his ball, safe and warm. Something that night led me back into the room with him.

Turning on the small lamp at the head of the bed, I positioned it sideways to dim its brightness. I turned off the blinding overhead light, and shut the door. I pulled the available chair closer to the stretcher where J lay, and sat down.

"Now what do I do," I thought. In the past my words — my talking — always seemed to aid a silence full of unanswered questions. So talk I did.

I don't recall all that I said or asked, but I know I shared with J about myself and my career in nursing, interlaced with questions about him, receiving replies of inhalations and exhalations.

On I talked and on he breathed.

One of the other nurses opened the door after a while and asked if I was okay. I nodded yes and asked her to bring me a cup of coffee with cream. J did not reply to my request if he wanted one as well.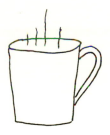

Anne whispered toward me, "What are you doing in here?"

"J and I are talking, Anne," I said. "We are sharing stories."

Being in the room with J for over an hour, I felt chilled in my short- sleeved white cotton shirt and pants. I was used to running all night, not sitting, yet I knew this was where I needed to be.

I retrieved two warmed flannels from the blanket oven, returning to tell J what I had brought. As I pulled down the thermal blanket, his left hand grabbed the edge of it, and hung on.

"J, I want to place a warmed blanket next to you with the other one on top."

He let me finish and when I sat down again with the other cozy warm flannel around my shoulders, I saw his body relaxing and his rigidness easing. I drank my coffee and spoke less, leaving great gaps of stillness. Funny, at times, I found myself matching my breathing pattern to J's.

The nursing staff assured me they would call if I was needed, so I continued to sit with him. When the physician returned to the department, the staff told him I had been speaking with J for more than an hour already. The doctor decided not to examine him at that time and returned to ICU.

My bum was sore, but I felt warmer as 2 a.m. clicked by on the broad-faced wall clock. I leaned back in the chair, placing my white-shoed feet against the side rail and, yes, you

guessed it, kept talking.

Some time later, I got up to go to the bathroom. I explained this to J and as I opened the door, he moaned. When I returned, I placed my hand on his shoulder, telling him I would be right back with a cheese sandwich that we could share. No response.

When I returned, I sat down, this time placing my hand on J's right arm. Within 20 minutes, I heard him sniffling and saw that he was crying. I left my hand where it was and kept talking.

The crying grew louder, becoming sobs with whole-body shaking. I sat quietly now and let his tears flow. Slowly J began to speak, mournful words and sad thoughts.

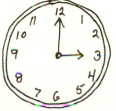
Coming on 3 a.m., J was focusing on me through the side rail bars as he delivered his story.

His crying lasted a long time. He refused tissues but wiped his nose with his sleeve and the blanket.

What I heard frightened me, shocked me and disgusted me, but I stayed. J grew angry and sat up at times shaking his fisted hand, gesturing with force. It was not directed at me, but at others in the world.

A knock at the door and it opened, Anne and the doctor peering in. "Everything okay in here? We heard noises."

"Yes," I replied and felt myself visibly shaking. "I will be out in a minute."

I offered J some juice and he quickly drank several small containers.

I left the room, the door ajar, and headed to the desk where I asked Anne to keep an eye on J while I spoke with the doctor in another room. I was shaking as I revealed some of J's history to the attending physician.

There were twists and turns that left my hair on end and my eyes bulging, as I grew as angry as J.

It is said that truth is stranger than fiction and that night I learned just how strange.

Retrieving another warm blanket to help myself stop shaking, I went back in with J. He no longer needed a blanket as he was warm with rage and release. J went on talking, letting out loud bursts of fury, and I kept listening. By 4 a.m. he became calmer. He ate a couple of sandwiches and had more juice and water.

J insisted on going home. He asked me to call one of his friends to come for him, and I did. The doctor never spoke with or examined him.

By 5 a.m. J was gone. He had shared his renewed life plan with me and I believed he would follow through with it.

The art and science within me married tightly that night,

allowing me to stay in that room with J. It guided me to talk or listen as needed.

I will never forget that night, and hope that J went on with his life as he had planned. I often wonder where he is and how he is doing.

Looking back, I realized that I had been in a place of acceptance of myself as a woman and a nurse during the winter that J arrived in the department. If I had not been accepting of myself I would not have stayed in the room with him. I would have judged him at the onset of his emergency visit and the outcome would have turned out a whole lot different.

As I blend the black and white of analysis and intuitiveness, I gain a wider grey area of unconditional acceptance. I have often waffled back and forth; now I merge them the best I can. This union heartily embellishes my nursing abilities. Analytical intuitiveness is easily displayed in the short minutes I spend with someone, or, when afforded the opportunity, allowed to serve over a lengthy period of time.

The most beautiful thing we can experience is the mysterious. It is the source of all true art and science.
Albert Einstein

Dear Flo,

I am writing for your advice on relationships. I do not know how
to come to terms with Science's lack of feelings.
Having brains is a wonderful attribute, but being
with a machine is not comforting.
Also, I feel overpowered and insignificant in the
presence of such intelligence, and am allowing
this to inhibit me. How can I get Science to open
up?

Art

Dear Art,

You can play a significant role by showing Science a healthy way
of being vulnerable. Courageously and respectfully sharing your
true feelings will create a foundation for Science to reciprocate.
Higher education does not necessarily breed humanistic
knowledge.
You are indeed two halves of the same apple,
both needed to create the whole. All brains or
all heart is neither healthy nor productive.
Together you will complement and
enhance each other, providing
a safe environment for growth.
With your forces joined, you will
embark on the true practice of
nursing.

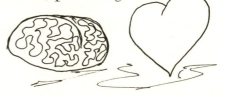

Ever yours,
Flo

Intimacy

"Intimacy is in-to-me-see."
Robert Burney

In the past, I was scared to let others in, my protective armor being miles thick. Believing that the world would not accept or love me as I truly was, I adopted fat as my most powerful defense.

I had numerous other shields, and keeping them intact and polished took a great deal of energy. Even in my marriage, I kept many layers strongly welded together. My armor shone, proudly portraying a satisfied wife, but I was not. I only showed the world what I thought they wanted to see.

I had lied to myself, my husband and everyone else about who I really was and how I truly felt. If I attempted to show the real me, I became angry and my words came out all wrong. I fluctuated from being a nice and perfect wife to being an angry helpless victim. I blamed my spouse but grew to understand that it was also very much my responsibility.

Instinctively, I knew if I showed my true self, I would have to leave the marriage. This truth festered under my security cloak, killing my emotions, my spirit, and my hopes and dreams.

I fell further and further into ugly despair, not knowing who I was, what I wanted or where I wanted to be. Hitting bottom, I ceased to feel.

I did not even know, let alone love, my authentic self, and I knew that she did not know how to love her husband. I was living a total lie.

It was in this self-dug hell-hole that I realized I needed to get to know myself. I began by searching everywhere for answers, most specifically within books and from talking with people I admired. Initially I gained back energy by changing words in my vocabulary.

Eventually I left my marriage, and today am still slowly letting go of my unhealthy ingrained beliefs. I am forgiving myself for past mistakes and accepting myself as hopelessly human. My defense shields are steadily disappearing, replaced by clear, healthy boundaries.

Now, I am intimate with myself, which allows me to be authentic with others. I have gained energy, and the realization of who I am and what I want is becoming clearer and clearer.

Someone told me a few years ago that I was honest to a fault. I thanked them, being proud of my accomplishment. Honesty is authenticity and authenticity is intimacy. These promote real life.

All this supports the marriage of my art and science within. Now, I am comfortable letting others know who I truly am and my writing clearly allows people this intimacy.

In the summer of 2005, I donated a copy of our first book for a convention's silent auction. The recipient of the book was the wife of a man attending the weekend gathering. This couple was staying in the same campground as I was and early that evening a truck pulled up by my site and out stepped a woman holding our book. She smiled as she came toward me, opening her arms to embrace me, and said, "I'm Sharon. I have only read part way through your book but I feel I already know you."

I smile as I realize how healthy being intimate is, not only for me but for everyone else.

Intimacy is reality, authenticity, love, friendship and relationship. It is healthy, real life and every human being is deserving of it.

As soon as you trust yourself, you will know how to live.
Goethe

Dear Flo,

Art is being so sensitive and emotional. This behavior drives me crazy mad, and when I tell Art to smarten up, I get blasted. I've even tried staying silent, but this also elicits a similar belligerent response. Why is Art so passive/aggressive?
I know I can be quite forward and stern at times ,but really, Art needs to chill out!

Seriously stern,
Science

Dear Science,

What is it about Art's behavior that bothers you? And why are you allowing it to get under your skin?
Other people's emotions often dictated my actions, feelings and thoughts, and I developed a vast array of knee-jerk responses.
As I grow more self respectful, I am able to ease these emotion-without-thinking responses and replace them with ones that are more logical, and respectful of us all.
When other people's communication is laced with emotional under and/or overtones, I look past the emotions, searching for what truly lies beneath.
I work to no longer react from my emotional place, and this gives them the respect that they deserve as a fellow human being. Their emotions do not persuade me to communicate from my own.
I know I can think and feel at the same time.
Often I will ask, " What do you need from me? What do you need me to do?"
Clearly stating and voicing these requests more than once grants others the opportunity to think beyond their emotional

outbursts. You are accepting them regardless of their behavior. This plain, respectful and unemotional communication allows the truth of their needs to surface.

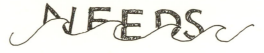

I have no right to tell others to stop crying, stop yelling or calm down ... these are their spontaneous reactions.
I can look past these to people's logic and receive a reply.
By doing this, I respect them as a human being.
I believe we each have triggers that set off the unconscious wounds of our past that sometimes control the way we act. In the moments when mine are prompted, I react better when someone accepts my presentation with no judgment; responding to the adult within me by asking what I need.
I recently learned the scientific reason behind this. When humans provoke and act from their emotional mid-brains and others respond to them from their own emotional mid-brains, the communication is ripe for staying stuck in the emotion. Thinking and logic come from our frontal lobe, and these are triggered by simple and respectful words.
When someone would arrive at the triage desk, loudly screaming, "I NEED HELP, #$%@*%$#@," I would often immediately reply, with a raised voice,"Stop that. Calm down or we won't treat you."

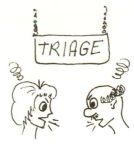

I judged and berated them and they, more often than not, reacted with further emotion. The conversation then frequently escalated to where I would threaten to — and would — call the security guard or the police.
If I had not displayed my knee-jerk reactions but had simply responded with, "Would you repeat that please?" or "What is

it that you need from me? What do you need me to do?" this would be communicating to their logical being. My calm, rational words would have eased their mid-brain emotions and respectfully elicited a quieter response. I have seen this to be true.

Science, you are learning — and allowing others — to think and feel, and therefore discover and promote the humanness in us all. Be patient with Art — and yourself.

Prone to passive/aggressive yet hopelessly human,
Flo

There Need to Be 'Is' in Team

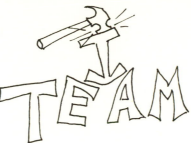

Remember always that you not only have the right to
be an individual, you have an obligation to be one.
Eleanor Roosevelt

Since my divorce, I have learned a great deal about
relationships. I've read book after book and devoured web
page after web page, wanting to understand what makes
personal unions tick and how to have successful ones. Although
I was seeking information about man/woman friendships, what
I garnered was enormous insight into the growth of healthy,
respectful and successful relationships of all kinds.

Teams are relationships,
and for healthy, respectful
and successful ones, each
person involved needs to be
encouraged to bring their
intimate, healthy self to the
table — their best 'I.'

Productive teams exist when individuals maintain themselves

as independent 'Is,' while working toward a successful 'we.' As each person garners the courage to voice their ideas, beliefs and boundaries in a respectful manner, and provides respectful receipt of these same things from others at the table, a win/win environment will exist.

What I have experienced, from both myself and others, is not this ideal.

When someone in the team gives up their 'I,' it leads to an unhealthy environment, fertile for autocratic management and a sense of hopelessness among those involved.

Several years ago, I was asked to attend a 'brainstorming' session for the implementation of an ongoing project. It was an exciting concept, one that I had been working on for many months. An urgent situation in the hospital forced me to be a half hour late for the meeting, which I was told would last for several hours.

I arrived apologetic and full of my ideas to share with those present. It became rapidly apparent to me that 'the plan' was already formulated.

Few of those in attendance were speaking; someone was dictating steps and another was writing them onto the chalkboard.

I challenged one of the developed ideas with what I viewed as a legitimate barrier for the successful process and outcome.

Silent stares, then, "Kathy, we need to push this through and it needs to de done now. We're behind on it."

Why was it called a brainstorming session if no such thing was to take place?

I realized that my energy had been wasted over the past months on ideas and problem-solving strategies for a project that I initially believed could have a favorable outcome. Now my enthusiasm for a successful conclusion was drowned out by gallons of self-serving silence. I sat through the remainder of the meeting not bothering to speak against anything proposed.

If I had been a stronger, more self respectful 'I,' the outcome may have been much more positive.

I missed the opportunity to muster the courage to be more persistently vocal with my ideas. Instead I walked away, choosing to do nothing further.

My best 'I' was not brought to that meeting.

What is learned can be unlearned. I can change myself.

Barbara De Angelis Ph.D., said, "Living a life of integrity means speaking your truth, even though it may cause conflict or tension; behaving in ways that are in harmony with your personal values; and making choices based on what you believe, and not what others believe."

Having visible and participating 'Is' leads to creative and successful problem solving. Each act of speaking and being heard yields a truly collaborative team.

I want 'Is' in my team because a team is stronger and more successful when the 'Is' are present. As I tame my nice nurse syndrome and heal my nerditis; as I marry my art and science and expose my leader within, I am more of an 'I.' This is who I take to meetings now; who I take into friendships now; and who I am.

Thou shalt not be a victim. Thou shalt not be a perpetrator. Above all, thou shalt not be a bystander.
Unknown

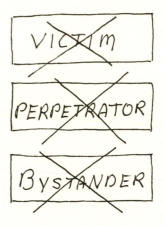

Dear Flo,

I am so passionate about myself and Science. These
strong desires interrupt my thoughts
throughout the day. Sometimes I am
driven crazy by all this zeal and it robs
me of sleep.
Oh, Florence what shall I do to calm myself? To not let myself
run away with my thoughts and feelings?
I feel like I am in a remake of The Taming of the Shrew.
How do I sit with my passion? How do I handle such enthusiasm?
How do I channel it wisely?

Rapturously yours,
Art

My strained Art,

If patience is a virtue, I so dearly need to practice my virtuosity.
I often jumped headlong into my passions, by writing and writing
and working and working. Now I see how unhealthy this was for
me.
If patience is passion tamed, then it is not the shrew
that requires taming, only the passion. With
subdued gentleness, I embrace my desires.
Art, I know you will keep your wits
about you and continue to live your
passions in a healthy manner. You are
already doing splendidly. I know you
will continue to tame and channel
your desires to your advantage.
Patience, persistence and time,

dear Art. Patience, persistence and time.

Yours truly,
Flo

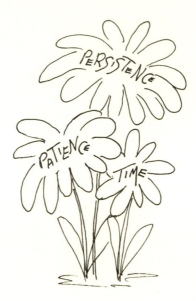

PPT — Patience, Persistence and Time

Patience and perseverance have a magical effect before
which difficulties disappear and obstacles vanish.
John Quincy Adams

In a world of instant tellers, fast food outlets and microwave popcorn, instant messaging, drive-by funeral body viewing and immediate lust leading to same-day love (well, some people's definition of love) ending in same-day sex, is it any wonder I need help learning patience, persistence and time (PPT)?

For me, PPT was unheard of, because I needed and wanted everything NOW!

I became an emergency room nurse because I enjoyed immediate responses and instant processing. My skills shone their brightest under fire and I prided myself on this accomplishment. I sped up, revved up and demanded top performance of myself. My fight or flight response was at its sharpest in high gear.

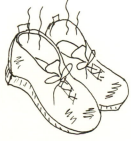

When I changed out of my duty shoes (runners), I remained fast paced in my personal life as well. I sped to get home to race through chores and multi-task life, working to provide everyone with instant gratification.

Isn't this what a good nurse, a good wife and a good mother should do?

Then my body and mind ground to a halt, forcing me to learn to be patient, to remain persistent and to embrace time.

I liken becoming knowledgeable in PPT to washing an **elephant**.

How does one wash an **elephant**?

One wipe at a time.

Will I go top to bottom or bottom to top? Front to back, back to front?

Pail, sponge, soap and water are readily available. A ladder may be helpful. No fancy high-tech-machinery is required, but plenty of elbow grease is advantageous at certain times.

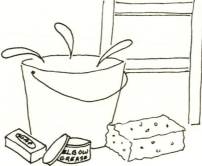

Do what you can with what you have where you are.
Theodore Roosevelt

I am cleaning the **elephant** a single wipe at a time, making my own choices. If one technique isn't satisfactory, I will try another and then another. I can re-decide.

Many times, though, I've wished it was a mouse to bathe — but alas, there before me is the **elephant**.

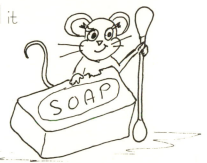

Previously viewing this as a foreboding task, I believed life was hopeless. Once I discovered my unlimited options, the laundering of the **pachyderm** became an enjoyable process. I've chosen to make a childlike adventure of it.

Sometimes, when I bite off more than I can chew, valuable lessons are learned. Stretching myself beyond my comfort zone allows me to experience life to its fullest. It is all in how I (eye) view the **loxodonta**.

"Moderation," said Oscar Wilde, "is a fatal thing. Nothing succeeds like excess."

In the past, I consulted numerous instruction books, seeking the perfect recipe — 'the perfect answer' — to my perceived **olifant** scrubbing dilemmas. Adopting other people's advice often caused me to become more confused.

Oh, what should I do? How should I do it? Would others approve of my choices? What is the 'right' way?

Sitting still and listening to my answers from within

provides me with the key to a jubilant washing of this enormous, childlike **mammoth**.

Interestingly enough, **elephants** communicate via infra sound — a long, slow-wave language, octaves lower than the human ear can detect. It is known as 'silent thunder.' These signals travel many miles, unaffected by obstructions. Scientist Katy Payne good-naturedly referred to them as 'long distance trunk calls.'

My inner voice is my infra sound communication and, with diligent attention, I can hear the answers.

The whole procedure is my responsibility; therefore, I can make different selections based on new information, even though others may criticize me.

I can make mistakes in this gigantic undertaking, learn from them and move on. For goodness sakes, it's only an **heffalump**.

Today, I am unsettled and scream for my personal changes and forward growth to happen right now! I want my dreams. I want. I want.

I am learning to be patient, but let's just get on with it!
Kathy Knowles

The **proboscidea** has reared its head, spraying me with water, and it is so HUGE at this moment. As I wipe my glasses to refocus, my alternatives become clearer. Reviewing the facts allows me to see that I have everything needed for this **elephantom** toilette and I gently remind myself of my overall vision.

Throwing a pailful of soapy water into the air, I say, "Why not? I needed a bath." Giggling and laughing, I can enjoy my silly ablutions.

Jumbo shrinks back to a manageable size because I am gaining the strength and courage to believe in my worth and value.

Once again, I am enjoying Snuffleupagus's bath one swipe at a time.

The Universe is concerned with who you are, and it will bring into your life, in whatever situations, in whatever time, what you need to become the person you're supposed to be. The key lies in trusting — having the patience.
Elisabeth Kübler-Ross and David Kessler

My life is living my dreams, moment by moment. The process of obtaining them is as relevant as the end reward. I am letting go to cherish and savor each step, each sponging of the **elephantidae**.

Letting go isn't giving up, it 's understanding that the best is yet to come.

Unknown

Patience, persistence and time is letting go. Will you bring your trunk(s) and join me?

To see the elephant (U.S. slang): to get experience of life, to gain knowledge of the world.

Oxford English Dictionary

Dear Florence,

I am out of sorts, restless and sad. As my relationship grows with
Art, I am feeling a loss. How can that be?
Am I scared that Art will run away from me? Is this it, my old
fear of abandonment?
I sense that it is different and yet the same, as if a part of me is
disappearing.
How can I be losing something as I grow in union with Art?
What do you suggest I do to ease my situation?

Grievously,
Science

Dear Science,

I believe that you are grieving the loss of your present. As you
grow closer to Art, you are shifting and changing parts of your
life: your time, your thought space, and possibly present routines.
Letting Art into your life is lessening your concentration on
yourself. Of course, you are feeling a sense of loss. This is
normal. We all fear the death of things, but it is those who can
embrace this life/death cycle that glean the greatest wealth —
knowing that after death follows life and as this wheel turns we
evolve as individuals. This is the way of the Universe.
We need to grieve our losses, allowing this reparative process to
take place. Welcome all the stages: denial, anger, bargaining,
depression and acceptance.[4] They will move you forward with an
appreciation for who you are becoming. Grieve and transform.
Congratulations, Science, you are doing splendidly. Believe in
yourself — in your courage — to work through the processes.
I believe in you and I believe that you can, will and are losing,
grieving and growing.

Meaningfully mournful,
Florence

Equality

To believe your own thought, to believe what is true for you in your private heart is true for all men — that is genius.
Ralph Waldo Emerson

When I allow competition to happen  between my art and science talents, I feel unsettled, and pulled apart. If I measure one against the other, one of them will be superior.

Am I a better nurse because I am smart or because I'm empathetic? Whom do I wish to emulate? Where do I belong?

I thought I was balancing the art and science of nursing and providing excellent patient care.

Our profession's widening scope of practice resulted in me being pulled to the science side. As a front-line nurse, I continuously updated my skills and education, with courses such as ACLS and TNCC, as well as in-house certifications. I counted on the educators in my area to provide the newest research information in such a manner that I could incorporate it into my practice.

Choosing to stay at the bedside while other nurses moved on with their formal education caused me to feel left behind, even though I

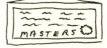

was constantly being tugged further into the science world. Attempting to do the 'splits' made me angry. My angst was directed at those who I thought were criticizing my choices, those involved in the science. Feeling threatened by other people's achievements also caused me to be angry toward myself. I realize that when I felt disenfranchised it was my lack of self respect showing.

If I concentrated on science, I neglected my art. I became distressed because I was straying from the nursing values I believe in: "the overriding concern and respect for the patient as a unique human being."

It saddens me that I allowed nursing advancements to cause an internal competition. I long for less dissension between the dualities of nursing. There is no need for this tug of war, because there is room for both within.

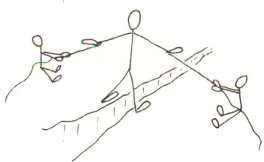

Let us value our training not as it makes us cleverer or superior to others, but in as much as it enables us to be more useful and helpful to our fellow creatures, the sick, who most want our help …

Florence Nightingale

When our first book came out, I was talking to a nurse who is working her way up the educational ladder. She said that she was proud of me and my co-author. Initially she had been upset and jealous, then became embarrassed when she realized that she had been viewing other people's achievements as competition. Once aware of this rivalry, she could dispel it and celebrate all nurses' accomplishments.

I was surprised and grateful for her disclosure. This colleague is ahead of the pack in her thinking. My respect for her grew in leaps and bounds that day and continues as I see her showing respect to others.

Conscious awareness and scrutiny of my art and science increases my self respect. I've stopped blaming the nurses who believe that increasing university education is our profession's answer to its credibility. It is my responsibility to give my artistic and scientific talents equal importance and I will do this by enhancing my self image and self worth. My advancements within our profession are from my own merit. Maintaining a cooperative art and science balance encourages excellence in nursing practice.

Treat people as if they were what they ought to be and you help them to become what they are capable of being.
Goethe

Tea and Sympathy

Art and Science arrive promptly at 2 p.m. and are ushered into a simple yet adequately furnished drawing room. They are directed to choose seating arrangements upon a lush emerald love seat and matching parlor chair. Science and Art choose the love seat and settle side by side.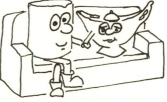

Florence sits in a stately rattan chair with overstuffed cushions. A wooden footstool is positioned within reaching distance of her feet. A woven shawl of natural-hued angora is draped across her knees. It is clearly her favorite place to sit, marked by a side table strewn with papers and books.

With a welcoming smile she says, "Thank you for coming. I wanted to share with both of you a few thoughts and stories regarding apathy, empathy and sympathy. These insights aided me in growing into a healthier and happier nurse and woman."

Silence, warm with anticipation, gathers in the room after her words, and Florence leans toward a glass-topped table to attend to the rituals of pouring tea.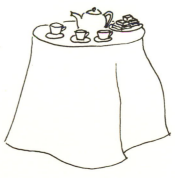

Flower-painted bone china cups

are filled with Orange Pekoe, and Science and Art each take one. Dainty cucumber sandwiches are served, and Art and Science settle in to listen to Florence's anecdotes.

Sitting back in her chair, leaving her tea cup perched on a paper pile,

Florence picks up a Webster's dictionary and begins to read.

"Apathy is a lack of emotion; lack of interest; indifference. Empathy is a capacity for participating in the feelings or ideas of others. Sympathy is a relationship between persons or things wherein whatever

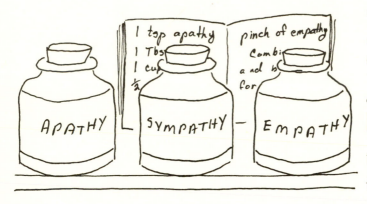

affects one similarly affects the others; compassion, pity."

Shutting the volume, she places it onto the floor.

"I was not taught in nursing school which of these stances to adopt — or if I was, I missed getting the message. Out of my intuitive motherliness I chose the act of sympathizing to begin my career. I took on other people's feelings and nourished them as my own, not realizing what this would do to me. My energy flowed to those in need and I took back their pain."

She pauses, taking a sip of her tea.

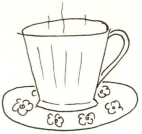

"The world's sorrows along with my own festered within me. I ached and hurt and slowly died inside. My heart and soul were a bundle of mis-shaped feelings and thoughts. I felt powerless to move beyond what was happening. As my energy lessened, I became angry and built walls to protect myself from the pain of others. Apathy wound tightly into my being and I lost interest in everything and everyone. I could not take on anything further and was lost within my tumultuous emotions, scrambling to climb back out into the world and failing miserably."

She shifts in her chair, offering more sandwiches to her guests, clears her throat and continues.

"Certain that I was the only nurse like this, I felt alone with my despair. I continued to shut down and turn off, scared to let others see me so ill because their eyes and mouths would judge as harshly as mine did.

Smarten up. Get a grip.

Don't be so silly about all this — just go for a walk.

I regularly trod marathons at work and at home.

Take up a new hobby.

I had way too many already.

Meet new people.

And what? Take on their stuff too? No, no way. I needed my energy reserves for my family, my work and for myself. I was trapped, and hated the apathetic woman in the mirror."

"My smiles were false as I struggled through my evening shifts at work. Home was a different story. I let out my anger there. It was my release and I showed it admirably while hiding all this from the world the best I could. I died inside, refusing to go back to being sympathetic. But was being held prisoner in apathy any better?

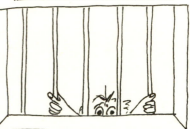

I felt hopeless and helpless and wanted to turn to someone, but each person I went to slammed me back down to my nothingness. They were no better off than I."

"An awakening came when I saw how poisonous the words 'I'm sorry' had become in my vocabulary. The judicious elimination of this simple phrase added great gains to my energy reserve.

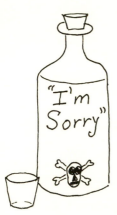

It has taken many years to continue my discovery and work on being empathetic. The simple awareness of the differences in these states of caring allows me to work at keeping my energy separate from others. I now have healthy boundaries of self protection.

Self awareness guides me toward empathy and I embrace it for health and happiness. I am stronger for the experience.

It is my responsibility to ensure my dominion — I am worthy of this respect. Believing in my worthiness allows me to believe in other people's abilities to carry their own load and feel their own feelings.

I will not take on anyone's stuff any longer. I will sit with and encourage them to trust their inner strength."

"This is not selfish. It is a healthy acceptance of my limits as a human being. The Universe does not want us to give ourselves away. It wants us to be fully who we are — true to our being. Practicing empathy allows me this choice."

"I choose empathy for self health, self worth, self fulfillment and self preservation. With this comes a healthier me to offer care to the world."

Florence stops to have more of her cooling tea. She motions to a small tray of petite fours. Both Science and Art decline.

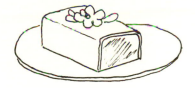

"Pity," she says. "They're homemade and very tasty."

She chooses one and savors its sugary, sweet goodness.

Upon completion, she speaks.

"It has been said that love is leading someone gently back to themselves. In the truest sense of the word, I, as a human being, love all others.

I can identify with other people's feelings without taking them on and can leave them where they reside, encouraging others in their self management. As I show others that they're capable of caring for their emotional needs, I am leading them gently back to themselves. This is empathy. This is love."

Art and Science appear deep in thought about this new-found knowledge of empathy.

"I know that you will make healthy choices for yourselves. Art and Science, I trust in your alliance and admire your courage to marry."

Florence embraces each of them as they take their leave.

The greatest good you can do for another is not just share your riches, but to reveal to him, his own.
Benjamin Disraeli

Goals For Me

I want to love you without clutching,
appreciate you without judging,
join you without invading,
invite you without demanding,
leave you without guilt,
criticize you without blaming,
and help you without insulting.
If I can have the same from you
then we can truly meet and
enrich each other.

Virginia Satir

The Dance

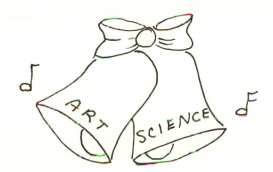

Marriage Announcement

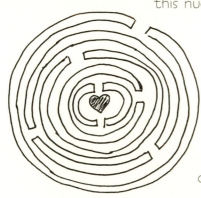

The official betrothal ceremony of Art and Science will be held in the 'practice' corridor connecting the Museum of Fine Arts and the Museum of Science.

An honor guard of trumpeters will flank the entrance and herald in the procession. Reflective lamplight will gently guide the footsteps of those in attendance.

A guest vocalist will grace the air with "Imagine," by John Lennon.

Art and Science will walk the marble floor's outlined labyrinth, which serves as a metaphor for their life journeys. Its path leads them to their souls' centers. A fusion within this nucleus signifies a movement toward a goal, allowing the release of emotions in order to create the united approach.

They will wear white uniforms and carry bouquets of olive branches and white roses intertwined with white flags.

   The flower girl and ring bearer will carry and disseminate
dozens of non-fragrant red roses, lengths
of ivy and pins of gold. Attendants have
chosen to don a combination of pastel,
white and green scrubs. Stethoscopes
will adorn their necks and they will carry
scentless blue forget-me-nots and babies'
breath. No mums allowed.

   All guests in attendance are required to wear backless
blue gowns and proper footwear. No slip-ons,
sandals or sling-backs, please.

   The spirit of numerous visionaries
will preside over the rituals: Mahatma
Gandhi, Leo Buscaglia, Buddha,
Abraham Maslow, Socrates, and
Florence Nightingale to name a few.

Art and Science will recite the Nurses' Declaration.

"With full awareness of the obligations we are undertaking,
   we promise to care for mankind with all the skill and
understanding we possess, without regard to gender, race, color,
politics or social status.

   We will keep our knowledge and proficiencies at the highest
level and share our wisdom, providing support to and cooperation

with all members of the health care team.

We resolve to make mistakes and learn from them, advancing toward excellence.

We vow to express our anger as appropriately as possible and encourage others to do the same.

We will cry, then support and sit with others as their tears flow.

We promise to find innocent humor each day, allowing others to hear our laughter and see us at play.

We pledge to recognize and ask for what we need.

We commit to advocate for ourselves and the patients, respectful of each other's dignities and beliefs.

We will practice forgiveness toward ourselves and then others, upholding the integrity of humanness."

These vows will be exchanged in all languages.

Humanistic nursing theorists will read the proclamation of their alliance, announcing them forever joined as Artistic Science.

Symbolic wreaths of orange blossoms, phlox and rosemary[5] will be placed upon their heads as they greet each other saying, "Namasté."[6]

Artistic Science will wind their way out of the soul-centering maze, accompanied by the recessional, "Can I have this Dance," by Anne Murray.

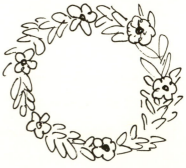

This sacred location will now and forever be known as the Hall of Humanness, where the Artistic Science of Nursing will be honored.

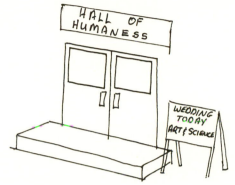

The Art and Science Song
(to the tune of "Love and Marriage")

Art and Science
Art and Science
Go together like
Trust and reliance
It's been rediscovered
You can't have one without the other

Art and Science
Art and Science
Need a pact of true alliance
Flo showed a truthful lead
You need to mirror this to succeed

Try, try, try
to keep them separate.
It's an illusion
Try, try, try, and
You'll arrive at this conclusion

Art and Science
Art and Science
Go together like
Trust and Reliance
It will stay uncovered
There can't be one without the other

Artistic Science
Artistic Science
Allows a humanness with no defiance
United, we are stronger
We can't stay apart any longer.

... Imagine The Future ...

Ideas are like rabbits. You get a couple, learn how to handle them, and pretty soon you have a dozen.
John Steinbeck

I believe it is time our profession moves forward to a place that creates an environment for nurses to examine and explore their own needs. Continuing to grow and learn about myself (my needs) allows me to remain in awe of the endless possibilities for my personal and professional life. As I imagine the exciting future that lies ahead:

I am certain that ideal patient care is through the soul;

I am certain that I will see a groundswell of nurses acknowledging and sharing their bountiful gifts;

I am certain that as self respect and acceptance spread, so will ideas;

I am certain that there will be non-punitive human resource policies in our health system;

I am certain there will be `emotion rooms´ for staff, as well as patients, to use;

I am certain there will be life coaches or counsellors devoted to staff in each facility;

I am certain the future holds a place for my dream,
in which there is a Canadian nurses' retreat for relaxing,
rejuvenating and rekindling spirits;

I am certain that I cannot imagine all the possibilities that
will be released when the ripple effect of increased self respect
takes hold within the health care system.

Ideal patient care is through the soul.

Spending many years going to workshops and taking
courses added to my nursing expertise; however, I neglected
the very knowledge that most affected patients in my care
— an awareness of myself.

I am now examining and acknowledging my feelings, the
when and why I have them. This leads to a full understanding
that how I feel affects how I react. This connectedness is
what I believe to be self awareness.

Increases in these inner alliances improve my relationships,
and the enhanced interactions cause positive health benefits
by decreasing my stress levels. I also experience less emotional
isolation, which reduces my chronic health issues.

The payoff for my inner reflecting is a healthier me, and
as a nurse, I am now more emotionally available to care for
patients.

It is taking time and energy to examine my past in order
to proceed into a healthier future. I feel saddened to

acknowledge how much more effective I could have been with my past nursing practice if I had been more self aware. I see self awareness as being in touch with my soul.

The strategies in my soul's tool kit are important for providing ideal patient care. My increased self awareness also reflects to those with whom I work.

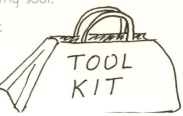

I believe an atmosphere of ideal patient care will grow out of a heightening of self awareness at every level within our health care system. Imagine what will happen when this ripple effect cascades outward.

Self acceptance and acceptance of others leads to new ideas.

Working together from a place of acceptance, I believe workplaces will become a safe, exciting environment for all to expose their creative ideas.

As I am becoming stronger and more accepting of my beliefs, I am sharing my ideas freely with others. My ideas are just that — ideas. They are not all that I am. If they are rejected, I recognize that this is not a rejection of me.

Health care systems have great potential that is tied closely to the people who come to work in them every day. If each person felt free to share their knowledge and ideas, imagine the possibilities for improvement.

I was recently chatting with a young porter while I awaited a minor surgical procedure. He was putting another stretcher beside me and I made a comment about the lack of space in the pre-op hold room. He gave me a quick response as to how the space problem could be easily fixed. I suggested he should pass on his idea, and he snorted, then said that he wasn't paid to think. 'They' weren't interested in what he had to say.

Even if this wasn't true, it was what he perceived to be true. What a waste of potential, what a waste of spirit. We went on to chat about places that offer incentives for staff input, places with proven track records of success, like Toyota, where respect and value are constant atmospheric components.

Hearing my thoughts echoed back to me from this young man helped me to know that Kathy and I are on the right path.

Respect and acceptance is the key to exposing new ideas. Imagine the future where there are no barriers to inventive concepts. As we celebrate the value of human beings, the rewards are limitless.

There will be non-punitive human resource policies in the health care system.

My nursing career, as well as my personal life, is full of contradictory messages.

"Don't think." versus "Use your head."

"You will work where I say." versus "As a professional you must know your limitations."

"Your sick time percentage is too high." versus "What are you doing at work spreading your germs?"

"Policies are guidelines, meant to be bent." versus "Legally you must follow policy."

As an employee, I am obligated to follow policies, protocols, guidelines and professional responsibilities. As a human being, I am often guided by my emotions. It is this human part that is causing my confusion.

It's no wonder I was in conflict with what to do when I was faced with a debilitating illness.

Taking time off, being on disability insurance and fighting with the insurance carrier about paperwork compounded my stress. Disagreements about collective agreement wording, especially about sick time, left me feeling undervalued as a person and an employee.

Assumptions, made by others, that I would know how to look after myself were wrong. Not only was I ignorant of the accessible services that would help me, most importantly I was unable to speak up for what I needed.

I came to the conclusion that I needed to take control and look after myself.

I believe that as human resource policies begin to allow

and to encourage nurses to take responsibility for themselves, without blame or shame, a healthier workplace will be created.

As local union president, I dealt with numerous return to work issues and sick time disciplines. Often I attended meetings where I believed there was judgment, disbelief, blame and shame leveled at the employee. I was, and still am, frustrated with many of the policies.

Because I was now owning my part in these meetings, I chose to begin a new relationship with the human resource representatives, using a straightforward and authentic approach. Clear, concise and respectful communication helped to steer most discussions away from the old blame-and-shame direction. Voicing needs helped to avoid confusion over what was expected from both sides. This respectful attitude was noted and returned by all parties, and I saw the treatment of nurses change.

As well, I diligently worked to impart to nurses that being ill or injured is not a character flaw, and that they are deserving human beings. I reminded them to be gentle with themselves, and, as I was learning to ask for my needs, I postured this to the nurses I worked with.

I strongly believe that the health care profession needs to advocate for improved relationships with all people, everywhere. Nowhere is this advocacy as important as within the halls of health care itself. I believe a supportive environment will enhance the growth and health of each individual employee. This investment in the staff is a value statement about their importance to the organization, now and in the future.

The health care system will reap the benefits of creating, and supporting, a healthier workforce.

There will be 'emotion rooms' for staff, as well as patients ,to use.

At present, I believe both nurses and patients are discouraged from showing their emotions

EMOTION
STATION

publicly and even privately. I am passionate about the creation of an environment that promotes emotional health. I support specific rooms set aside for that purpose alone.

These will be available around the clock, much like a chapel. The rooms need to be multi-functional: a corner conducive to comfort and relaxation, with a supply of Kleenex and cozy blankets. Another area with the availability of a 'whack a mole' game, punching bag, foam bats, or anything that could be used as an outlet for frustration and anger. I envision writing materials, humor books, magnetic poetry and a stereo with headphones.

To allow for the expression of all human feelings, without judgment, fosters an environment of well being.

Nurse-specific life coaches or counsellors will be in each facility.

In the future there will be life coaches available for nurses. Their focus will be on personal health and well being, inviting and supporting gentle self exploration.

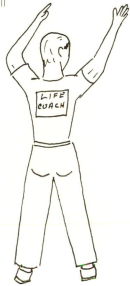

Even though I have supportive friends, there are times when I want an outside opinion, a verification that I'm on the best track for myself. Sometimes I need to unload, to a person who would not judge or rescue me. This is the life coach, someone who shows me my inner strengths and wisdom. Someone who is simply there.

I believe it is imperative for a healthier health care system that there be a coach/counsellor available for nurses on an ongoing basis. Being on-site will allow these coaches to build trusting relationships. I know most health regions have employee assistance programs already, but I see the difference being in the ease and comfort of access.

The opportunity to find trusted support in a facility is a win/win situation. Imagine the future where the focus is on nurses as human beings: a whole — body, mind and spirit.

The future holds a place for my dreams …

I visualize a retreat created for, and catering to, us 'contemporary' nurses. A place where we can learn to 'be,' in a comfortable, and accepting environment. Webster's New Explorer Dictionary and Thesaurus describes 'contemporary' as related to advanced: educated, enhanced, enlightened.

My imagination has taken me on a journey to this retreat in the Gulf Islands. A lodge made of cedar logs, with one 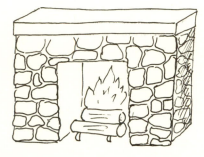 entire wall a stone fireplace. From the great room, I will look out over the water. The main floor will also include a large dining area, conference room, library and gourmet kitchen. Bedrooms for the caretakers will be upstairs in the loft, and guests will be in individual log cabins with ocean views.

You'll never succeed beyond your wildest dreams unless you have some wild dreams.

John L. Mason

This rejuvenating centre will provide opportunities for nurses to explore and celebrate their inner talents. Opportunities for music, art, golf, poetry, ocean adventures and silence will flow. The list is endless. I am enjoying the long walks, canoe rides and warmth from conversation by the wood-burning fireplace.

Imagine the benefits to health care as we contemporary nurses care for ourselves. This venture is more than possible and will be a reality. I know this is achievable, for I believe in myself and I believe in you.

These are my dreams at the moment, and I am working toward them. I will meet you at the water's edge one day soon. Imagine the

future . . .

If we wait for the moment when everything, absolutely everything is ready, we shall never begin.

Ivan Turgenev

Dear Florence,

Thank you for the support and guidance that you endowed
upon us during our path toward marriage. We appreciate your
friendship and belief in us, as individuals and as a united
influential power.

To celebrate our upcoming nuptials, we had an intimate dinner in
a field of wildflowers and tall grasses. This reminded us of Rumi's
words, "Out beyond right doing and wrong doing there is a field,
I'll meet you there."

What a splendid evening! Art
provided chairs and a small round
table, complete with a creatively
embroidered tablecloth. A glowing
lamp illuminated the event, blown
out only twice by the warm westerly
winds. Oh Flo, the music that those strong breezes made,
moving among the grass stalks sounded as if a string orchestra
was playing all around us.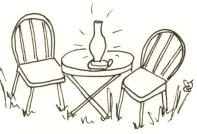

Science supplied beakers of wine and we dined on local cuisine.
There was no eating crow, as we now understand and accept the
frailties of our humanness.

A lively discussion took place about the powerful washing the
elephant piece. Patience, persistence and time allow us to discover
our answers within. While scrubbing our elephants the solutions
to our problems appear and, with courage, we put them into
practice.

Our individual remedies may be very different, but the outcome
is the same. Problems are solved and all problems are solvable. No
more grinning and bearing things. No more sucking it up and
stuffing it down.

Everyone needs to wash the elephant their way. If they ask for advice then it can be given, otherwise we need to stay silent and respect other people's inner knowledge. Unsolicited advice is disrespectful.

Florence, we laughed and cried, agreeing on certain topics while agreeing to disagree on others. This variance allows each of us to learn from a different perspective. Oh, what a marvelous best friendship we have.

In marriage, we will each remain independent thinkers while growing to a culminating voice. This will take work and unconditional love. We are prepared for the undertaking — an adventure that will advance the practice of professional nursing. Encouragement of each other to be our best is ultimately affecting the greater good of the sum. With this empowerment the Artistic Science of Nursing is sure to rock.

As we unite we become three

Art, Science and We.

RN pins were exchanged under the stars, a perfect ending for the evening of our beginning.

We look forward to meeting you in the Hall of Humanness.

Ever yours,
Artistic Science

My dear Science,

You know, an elopement would have been so much easier.

All this talk of cakes, caterers and commitment has me so confused.

I have a 30-foot ladder that would work beautifully to reach your windowsill. I envision us now, at dusk, out of other people's view. You with your beakers safely packed in a suitcase with evidence-based practice theories tucked in around them.

Intuitively, I would sew a nice little bag in
which to hold my empathy, listening ear
and creativity. Our stethoscopes would
tie everything together.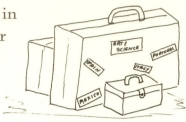
Oh, Science, come away with me
to a world of grace, forgiveness,
authenticity and caring. We will gain humanness while letting go
of perfection. We will become as one . . . Artistic Science forever.
There's room for us both.
This is the world we need. This is coming home.
Let's not wait another minute.
Will you dance this dance with me now?

With love and certainty,
Art

RSVP

Welcome, with your polished lamps ablaze.
Would you like to dance?
Will you dance?
When will you dance?

Awareness guides the shameless waltz of full acceptance
Courageous boundaries clearly marked.

Trust with appreciation while
Forgiveness and empathy pave the way.
Answers lie within, distinct yet connected.
Unique steps will be approved.

Feelings take the floor, knowing
Patience, persistence and time are all there is.
That's all there is my friend
So let's start dancing.
Let's shed aloof and have it all.

The music sways us to true believing.
Let's start receiving vows of friendship.
With ladder placed against the window
Science joins with Art, as one.

This simple showing will cause a growing.
Artistic Science please lead on.

Dancing is the last word in life ... in dancing one draws
nearer to oneself.

Jean Dubuffet

P. I. F.
Permissions, Interests and Forever Grateful

Linda and Kathy thank the following publishers and authors who gave permission to reprint writings from their selected works.

"As we approach a new...." from *The Sacred Balance: Rediscovering Our Place in Nature,* pp.55, David Suzuki, 1997, Published by Greystone Books, a division of Douglas & McIntyre Ltd.. Reprinted with permission from the publisher.

Goals For Me, from *Making Contact*, pp.194, Virginia Satir, 1976, Celestial Arts, a division of Ten Speed Press, Berkeley, CA. www.tenspeed.com. Reprinted with permission from the publisher.

Reasonable attempts were made to trace the original sources of quotes and concepts within this book. If errors or omissions are found by copyright holders, please contact the publisher.

Endnotes:

1. **artistic science**, pp.27, is a creation based on the word 'art-science' from <u>Humanistic Nursing Practice Theory</u> by Loretta Zderad PhD and Josephine G. Paterson PhD.

2. **mad, sad, glad and scared (fear)**, pp.99, are considered the four basic feelings. The knowledge of this concept was obtained while attending a Transactional Analysis (TA) psychology workshop.

3. the **Drama Triangle**, pp.130, is psychiatrist Dr. Stephen Karpman's diagram for analyzing social games. It displays the roles that we 'act-out' in our daily lives.(Rescuer, Persecutor and Victim) The TA world describes these roles as 'unstable, unsatisfactory, repeated and emotionally competitive, and they generate misery and discomfort, sooner or later.' People caught in triangular games have no healthy limits nor do they use enough words to describe or solve problems.

4. the stages of grief: **denial, anger, bargaining, depression and acceptance**, pp.185, are those described by Elisabeth Kübler-Ross.

5. **orange blossoms, phlox, rosemary:**, pp.198, orange blossom signifies eternal love and marriage; phlox signifies united souls; and rosemary represents love, loyalty and friendship.

6. **namasté**, pp.198, is a South Asian greeting meaning: I honor the place in you where Spirit lives. I honor the place in you which is of Love, of Truth, of Light, of Peace. When you are in that place in you, and I am in that place in me, then we are One.

Books that influence us:

Brammer, Lawrence M., *The Helping Relationship Process and Skills*, Prentice-Hall Inc., New Jersey, 1973.

Burney, Robert, *Codependence: The Dance of the Wounded Souls*, Joy to You&Me Enterprises, California, 1995.

Buscaglia, Leo, *Loving Each Other: The Challenge Of Human Relationships*, SLACK Inc., New Jersey, 1984.

Clarke, Jean Illsley, *Self-Esteem: A Family Affair*, Harper Collins Publishers, New York, 1978.

Compton's Pictured Encyclopedia, volumes 1-9, F .E . Compton & Company, Chicago,1925.

Donahue, M. Patricia, PhD, RN, *Nursing: The Finest Art,*

C.V. Mosby, *Missouri,* 1985

Evans, Dylan, *Emotion: The Science of Sentiment*, Oxford University Press Inc., New York, 2001.

Goleman, D., PhD, *Emotional Intelligence*, Bantam Dell, A division of Random House Inc., New York, 2005.

Goleman, D.; Boyatzis, Richard; and McKee, Annie, *Primal Leadership: realizing the power of emotional intelligence,* Harvard Business School Publishing, Boston, 2002.

Joines, Vann and Stewart, Ian, *TA Today: A New Introduction to Transactional Analysis,* Nottingham and Chapel Hill Lifespace Publishing, 1987.

Jones, Laurie Beth, *The Path,* Hyperion, New York, 1996.

Kübler-Ross, Elizabeth and Kessler, David, *Life Lessons*, Schribner Publishing, New York,2000.

Mason, John L., *Let Go Of Whatever Makes You Stop*. Insight International, Oklahoma, 1994.

Merriam-Webster, *Webster's New Explorer Dictionary and Thesaurus* New Edition, Federal Street Press, a division of Merriam-Webster Incorporated, Massachusetts, 2005.

Mintzberg, Henry, *Managers not MBA'S*, Berrett-Koehler Publishers, Inc., San Francisco, 2004.

Morrison, Andrew P. MD., *The Culture of Shame*, Ballantine Books, New York, 1996.

Peale, Norman Vincent, *Norman Vincent Peale's Treasury of Courage and Confidence,* Double Day & Company, New York, 1970.

Pierce, R.V. M.D., *The People's Medical Adviser In Plain English or Medicine Simplified*, World's Dispensary Medical Association, New York, 1914.

Satir, Virginia, *Making Contact,* Celestial Arts, a division of Ten Speed Press, California, 1976.

Smith, Manuel J., Ph.D., *When I Say No I Feel Guilty,* Bantam Books, New York, 1975.

Suzuki, David, *The Sacred Balance: Rediscovering Our Place In Nature*, Greystone Books, a division of Douglas & Mcintyre Ltd.,Vancouver, 1997

Vicinus, Martha and Nergaard, Bea, *Ever Yours, Florence Nightingale: Selected Letters*, Virago Press, Great Britain, 1989.

Vincente, Kim, PhD., *The Human Factor*, Alfred A. Knopf Canada, a division of Random House Of Canada Limited, Toronto, 2003.

Watson, Lyall, *Elephantoms: Tracking the Elephant*, W. W. Norton & Company Inc., New York, 2002.

Wilber, Ken. *The Marriage of Sense and Soul: Integrating Science and Religion*, Broadway Books, a division of Random House Inc., New York, 1998.

Woodham-Smith, Cecil, *Lonely Crusader: The Life of Florence Nightingale 1820-1910,* McGraw-Hill Book Company Inc., 1951.

Zukav, Gary, and Francis, Linda, *The Heart of the Soul: emotional awareness,* Simon and Schuster, New York, 2001.

Websites that are a source of wisdom:

wwww.en.wikipedia.org
www.ta-tutor.com
www.joy2meu.com
www.ahpweb.org
www.cna-aiic.ca
www.humanisticnursingtheory.com
www.claudesteiner.com

As our journey continues toward an acceptance of ourselves as hopelessly human we wish to thank:

Betty Kendall for her friendship, wisdom and inestimable guidance.

Rosalie Wilson for her creativity, talent and support.

Yvonne Jeffery for her valuable input and editing.

Dave and staff at The Warwick Printing Co. Ltd. who are there each step of the way.

And to our friends at the main postal office in Lethbridge for their smiles and ongoing support.

Thank you to those who believe in me and extra thanks and love to Bryan for his presence in my life. My family and friends continually support and assist me, and for this I am grateful. Linda consistently and faithfully believes in what we are doing and I am thankful for this along with her patience, acceptance, and ongoing immersion in this amazing adventure.

K.K.

With my heart full of gratitude and love I say thanks to Kathy, my friend and co-author for her patience, persistence and time.

Love and thanks go to my family and friends. Your support and love sustain me.

To my extended work family, thank you. My spirit is nourished by your encouragement and belief. Together, we are tilting the direction of health care.

L.B.